Why Don't You Drink Alcohol?

101 Reasons To Stop Drinking Like A
Woman Called Karen And Why Sobriety Is
The Key To Unleashing Your Best Self.

Quit Lit For Women.

By Sienna Green

A Little Poem About Alcohol:

It starts with just a sip or two
But soon it gets its claws in you
You lose control and all your might
Fall victim to its hypnotic sight.

Your body aches, your mind is dull
You're trapped inside a drunken lull
The morning after leaves you weak
As you search for what you cannot seek.

But there is hope, a brighter way
To live life with joy each day
Embrace sobriety, let it shine
And watch your life transform divine.

Clear eyes, a peaceful mind
The path to bliss you'll easily find
Sober living, it's the key
To unlock life's true majesty.

Abandon the bottle, take a stand
Become the master of your own brand
Sobriety will set you free
From the chains of alcohol's misery.

Live life with meaning, purpose and zest
With love and joy, not booze as a guest
Say no to the tempter's call
And embrace sobriety for all.

(If you relate to this poem, strap yourself in for the rest of the book!)

Table of Contents

INTRODUCTION

I'm not qualified to write this book.

Not in the traditional sense, anyway. I'm not a doctor. I'm deeply interested in human psychology and what makes us who we are, but at best, I'm an 'armchair psychologist.'

I'm not an academic, either. I apparently have a theatre degree, but I was too busy riding my full-blown journey off the rails to attend the graduation ceremony (really).

What I do have is a decade of humiliation, horror stories, and hangovers. I was an alcoholic from the moment I picked up my first drink. Moderation was never even a possibility. From that first Vodka Cruiser when I was around eighteen, I was a habitual binge-drinker. It was so unconscious, so automatic, as though I never even thought I had a choice in how I consumed.

We're conditioned from childhood to look forward to being able to drink. Alcohol is the elixir of adult life. It's romance, parties, sporting events, and great times with friends. It's a rowdy round of beers with your best friends at the pub, a popped champagne bottle to celebrate an engagement, or a glass of red wine at an elegant, candlelit dinner table. It's sugary cocktails with miniature umbrellas by the pool on vacation. It's American movies with people playing beer-pong and guzzling out of red cups. These images are indelible to us. They're also, for the most part, a horrible lie.

Alcohol wreaks havoc on your body and mind. Alcohol abuse is a common, debilitating, and chronic condition.

If you're reading this, I assume you are newly sober, sober-curious or just looking for reminders as to why you gave it all up in the first place. Perhaps you wish to quit drinking temporarily just to see how you feel. Maybe you want to support a friend, partner or relative in their sobriety. Perhaps you've hit your idea of 'rock bottom' (I hit about twenty of those before I finally said enough was enough), and you need some encouragement and motivation for the journey ahead.

Admitting that alcohol has become a problem for you, or even that you suspect your life would be better without it, can be immensely challenging. You're probably surrounded by people who drink, and some of them may be threatened by you quitting. They'll give you shit. They'll buy drinks on your behalf and mock you mercilessly until you cave in. You'll realize you're never too old to be relentlessly peer pressured!

This book exists for your mental fortification. Within these pages, I will lay out 101 reasons why you should stop drinking alcohol (we will get to the 'Karen' bit later), or if you've already quit, why you should stick with it. It's not going to take all 101 reasons to convince you. I'm sure of that. Some of these facts are brutal and confronting. Some of them will shock you. I was certainly floored many times by what I learned throughout my research. As a non-academic, non-doctor, total layman, I couldn't believe everything I hadn't been told about alcohol. I'm not advocating prohibition here, but shit.

This stuff does so many terrible things to your body, brain, relationships, career prospects, family, and basically every aspect of life you can think of. We might have heard vague warnings about carcinogens, but there are vague warnings about carcinogens on pretty much everything, right? I mean, we've all just kind of accepted that modern life is slowly (or rapidly, depending on where you live) poisoning us all, haven't we? So why not chug down a little of the poison that *at least* makes us feel good in the moment and helps us forget about it all? I get it. I feel like a drink right now, thinking of the vast horrors of the world, and it's 9:35 am, and I've been sober for seven years. But after you read these facts, you will want to protect yourself. You will understand that imbibing something that is so across-the-board awful for you is not worth it for the temporary buzz, the brief, illusory feeling that comes right at the beginning of the night, before, if you're anything like me, you either descend into the depths of your buried despair or have horrible sex with someone you will be gravely repulsed by in the harsh light of the morning sun.

Drinking culture is a beast. I'm an Australian; I get it. We get pissed. We get blotto. We get cunted (a personal favorite). We get, inexplicably, 'maggot.'

When the personal demons that caused me to drink so hard and fast intersected with a culture that actively encouraged overconsumption, you get the decade that was my twenties. So that's what brings me here. From my first drink around 18 to my final drink on my 29th birthday, I was addicted to binge drinking. Again, it wasn't like there was one particular event or incident that made me realize I had to stop. I'd had so many things happen in my decade of drinking that *should* have been the end, that perhaps *would* have been the end for someone more reasonable. It was the accumulation, the weight of those ten years of daylight shame, and the understanding somewhere in the blocked-out recesses of my mind that this was not the life I was supposed to be living. That this couldn't be it. That something had gone very wrong.

In sobriety, I have gained insight from years of trying to figure out how to give myself the self-love and self-esteem I never got from a healthy home life. I spent years facing all that I was trying to block out with the binging behaviour. And I have seen through the facade of the alcohol companies who try to convince us through their insidious advertising and marketing campaigns that life is better when alcohol is at the center of it.

It isn't. I can say with no falsity that I love being sober. I love not waking up with a parched mouth and a beam of sunlight boring directly into my eyes, with those few confused moments of not knowing where I am quickly giving way to a dawning horror as I remember the humiliating things I said or did. I love not spending the entire next day in bed with a screaming headache, interrupting my groaning and feeling sorry for myself, only to go to the bathroom and attempt to retch up whatever's left in my stomach. I love not finally rousing myself at 6 pm when my nausea has passed and then treating myself to a Macca's binge to commemorate another wasted day. I love that I can go to a friend's birthday celebration, completely control my faculties, and remain lucid and self-aware. I love to have conversations that I can actually remember. And I love that I can leave when people start getting sloppy and close-talking and be cuddled up safely in my bed by 11 pm. I can wake up the following morning feeling optimistic, have my first cup of coffee while reading or journaling, take a long hike, clean my apartment and still have time and energy left in the day. I am fully lucid and present for every moment of my life. I am a participant. I can't imagine wanting to feel any other way.

Of course, I didn't feel this way immediately. It took some time to love being sober. Stripped of the thing I always used to hide behind, that I always buried my insecurities in, I flew headlong into all the anxieties I'd been covering up. I could no longer hide. I had no crutch in social situations. I had to face the idea that I might hate myself or that, at the very least, I didn't really know how to like myself.

The truth was, I had no idea who I was. When I was growing up, I loved reading and was thrilled whenever a school assignment involved writing. I didn't have a problem making friends. I felt confident and certain of my position as a valuable part of the world. I've heard that a lot of young girls feel this way before the various horrors of puberty descend and they become hyper-aware of how people see them, and whether people think they're pretty or chubby or their clothes are cool enough. The feeling of self-love and being sure of your place in the world doesn't often survive that onslaught, unless you have a strong support system. And in the parlance of my country, yeah nah, I didn't have that.

My mother had always been prone to extreme emotional swings and fits of rage, and her mental condition began to deteriorate further in the years following her divorce from my father when I was about 4. He remarried and found happiness with a very sweet woman, and my mother's anger at him for not just sticking around to endure her tantrums grew yearly. I was too young to remember when her abuse towards my brother and me began, but it intensified in the years following the divorce. She wouldn't just scold us for our childish mistakes. She would scream and scream until her voice was strained, her vicious tirades sometimes going on for hours. She would push us against walls and slap our faces over minor mistakes. She said cruel and insulting things to us, and sometimes a smile would creep over her face as she did so. I mean, the word sadist seems like *a lot* when describing one's mother, but I'm not sure what else to call an adult woman who smiles while hurting a child's feelings. She mocked us when we cried, and if we ever dared say *anything* in response to her haranguing, even just to try to explain ourselves, she'd accuse us of 'attacking' her. Incidentally, anyone who disagreed with her was accused of 'attacking' her. She told strangers and acquaintances how proud she was of her family, and then, as soon as the front door closed, she became our tormentor. She took credit for any tiny victory we had, be it an academic award or a compliment from an outsider on our manners, but any small mistake we made was because we were inherently stupid, useless, and pathetic, three of her favorite words.

Although I was usually in the 'gifted' classes in primary school, I had become utterly numb about my studies by high school. I withdrew socially. I mainly lived in my head, where I concocted elaborate fantasies about being someone talented, world-famous and adored. Despite my palpable shyness, I dreamed of being an actress, and after I'd managed to finish high school, I was accepted into a theatre program at a university. This was completely unexpected, as I thought I'd done terribly in the audition. Perhaps they saw something beneath my insecurity that they thought could be channelled into a character. But I was never able to break through. I'd been taught to suppress my emotions by my mother. "Stop crying, or I'll give you something to cry about" was her favorite (and highly unoriginal) expression. I started drinking heavily during the three-year program. I lived in a shabby house with four classmates, working in a discount store part-time to barely afford my share of the rent and making important daily decisions like whether to spend my last $5 on coffee, a loaf of bread or a cheap bottle of wine. The booze usually came out victorious (the drink itself was the only thing victorious). No one thought I was a young Meryl Streep, but I made it through the course with a whimper, thinking more about the after-party of our final performance than the industry professionals who had come to watch and assess us. As a final insult to my ambitions, I blew off the graduation ceremony.

Despite my best efforts, I actually received an offer of representation from an agency, who burdened themselves with the thankless task of trying to find me work. I drank before auditions to 'calm my nerves' and then showed up still very nervous but also erratic, sweaty, and liable to forget every one of my lines. I partied when I should have been preparing. Drinking gave me an excuse for failing at what I claimed were my dreams. The period from eighteen to twenty-nine was typified by unfulfilled potential, self-destructive behaviour, poor choices, and trying to quiet the anxiety and perpetual undercurrent of impending doom that had been with me since childhood.

How I wished I could stop at one or two. It never happened. Not even once. I wasn't actively trying to ruin my life every time I had a night out. If I could have stayed in the relaxed buzz zone, I would have. But I would inevitably keep going. There was no off switch.

And then there was my drinking buddy Karen. You might know a 'Karen', you might even be that 'Karen', but one thing is certain, alcohol and 'Karens' don't mix. Alcohol was terrible for me, I don't deny that, but it can always be a shit tonne worse for someone else. Alcoholics Anonymous taught me to look at the 'similarities and not the differences' regarding other people and their drinking. Still, sometimes you just can't ignore it because their allergic reaction to alcohol cause ripples of chaos that impact many people. The benefits of sobriety are for everyone, Karen, me and anyone with a relationship with alcohol.

I had so many points of rock bottom that it's hard to pinpoint what made me finally decide to 'take a month off'. What happened to Karen was certainly one BIG factor because it made me take some time to reflect on my relationship with alcohol (that life-altering incident is discussed later). It was just another impulse at the time. I'll try this sobriety thing out. I wasn't in touch with my inner voice yet. That voice that, if you sit quietly by yourself for long enough, meditate, or take a walk in silence, you can access, however briefly. That deep inner knowing behind the clatter and chatter of your mind, all the myriad distractions. Maybe somewhere buried under all my nonsense, I knew my path was one of misery and that I would never become the person I wished to be if I didn't stop. So it made a deal with my conscious mind; let me believe this is just for a month.

I'm trying something out. That month became three, and after three months, I knew it was forever. But there was pain too. I had to begin navigating the world without my crutch. Without the chaos that drinking caused, I had nothing to distract my thoughts. Without regrets, arguments, and dealing with the fallout of my big nights, life became very quiet. And then the thoughts arose. I found myself having to confront intensely painful memories of my childhood. Memories surfaced of instances I hadn't thought about in years. I understood why I drank so hard and fast every time. I was seeking a sort of obliteration, to completely forget who I was and everything I couldn't stand about myself.

I bring you this guide not because I'm some kind of professional but because I'm certainly not. In relatively simple and straightforward terms, I aim to present some facts about alcohol that have helped me stay the course of my sobriety. These things remind me whenever I feel tempted to see if, after all this time, I can become the kind of person who "just has one or two", that it's not worth it. Beyond the humiliations and hangovers, alcohol is terrible for your body, and alcohol abuse devastates individuals, families, and society. If you're thinking about giving up alcohol, I hope that something you read in this guide might give you the final push you need. If you've already quit and need encouragement to stay on track, I hope you'll find all the sobering (sorry) information you need right here.

Before we get into the 101 reasons, it is critical to mention that quitting alcohol "cold turkey" can be extremely dangerous for certain people. If you're a frequent or heavy drinker, it may lead you to experience symptoms like nausea, insomnia, shaky hands and headaches, and life-threatening outcomes such as seizures, hallucinations and hypertension. If you believe you may have a physical dependency on alcohol, please take the time to consult with a medical professional before you commence your sober journey.

I'm betting that you'll be convinced after about ten of these (at least!). If you relate to more of this book than you would like to admit, take it as a sign that giving up alcohol might be the best thing you ever do. And no, I won't buy you a beer if I'm wrong.

REASONS 1-19

- YOU CAN'T IGNORE THESE (BUT YOU KEEP IGNORING THEM ANYWAY)

These reasons are precisely why it's worth considering giving up alcohol. You've likely overlooked them by justifying that drinking "isn't that bad."

However, as you progress through this chapter and the following ones, you may find yourself re-evaluating that perspective entirely.

1. PASSING OUT IS MORE DANGEROUS THAN YOU THINK

From the time I had my first drink at around age 18, I seemed unable to moderate my consumption. Once I was intoxicated, there was no conception of an off-switch. I didn't stop until I passed out, whether that was in my bed (the ideal scenario), a stranger's bed (reasonably likely), or sometimes right where I was, even if that was the filthy, cold tiles of the bathroom of the bar. I will be forever grateful that I have always regained consciousness.

Alcohol overdoses occur when there is more alcohol in the bloodstream than the body can process. It can lead to the essential functions of life-support, such as breathing, heart rate, and temperature controls, shutting down. It becomes perilously easy to choke on your own vomit. In the worst-case scenario, permanent brain damage or death can occur.

This scenario is hazardous when coupled with the misconception that someone who has passed out can be left to just 'sleep it off.' Don't believe the movies: the worst thing that could happen ISN'T that you could wake up with a cornucopia of dicks drawn on your face.

As just one of many tragic examples, the iconic AC/DC band member Bon Scott died at 33 after being left to 'sleep off' his drunkenness in a friend's car following a night out.[1] This is a remarkably easy mistake to make in the moment, especially considering the detrimental effect that alcohol has on the decision-making processes of the prefrontal cortex, a part of the brain you'll be hearing a lot more about as we move through the 101 reasons why you might want to stop drinking.

As you will see later, when we discuss 'that' incident with Karen, it only takes that one time. It might not have happened to you all those other times, but what happens if it happens next time?

2. PEOPLE ALMOST NEVER TREAT A PASSED-OUT PERSON CORRECTLY

Medical professionals recommend that passed-out people be woken up every 5-10 minutes and checked for signs of alcohol poisoning. The reason is that, for the first hour of being passed out, your body *continues* to process the alcohol already consumed. That means that your blood alcohol concentration (BAC) can still increase, even while you're asleep.

For reference, and in case you find yourself in the position of monitoring someone else, signs of alcohol poisoning encompass the following:

- Confusion
- Vomiting
- Seizures
- Slow breathing
- Inconsistent breathing
- Skin turning blue or ashen skin
- Low body temperature
- Inability to be awakened[2]

Hypothetically speaking, what do you think the chances are of a person who is passed out at a party being monitored safely? Especially when they're surrounded by other drunk people? The 'let them sleep it off' fallacy is all too common.

Even if you're lucky enough to have a friend or partner who has the awareness to monitor you in your passed-out state, you probably aren't going to feel great about burdening them by placing your fragile and precious life in their hands all night. People who regularly become intoxicated to this extent put extreme physical and emotional strain on their friends and family. Having to constantly protect someone you care about from the fallout of their own poor choices is profoundly draining. It can lead to relationship resentment, which we will discuss in greater detail as we progress.

3. THE ABJECT HORROR OF BLACKOUTS

The term 'blacking out' is sometimes used interchangeably with 'passing out', but the two states are distinct. While passing out refers to losing consciousness due to drinking too much, blacking out is when an intoxicated person is physically awake, but their brain is not processing the events that are occurring or creating new memories.

Blackouts happen when alcohol causes the brain to temporarily halt its 'memory consolidation' function. Taking place in the hippocampus, this involves the transfer of short-term memories to long-term storage. Blackouts are more inclined to occur when blood alcohol concentration (BAC) reaches 0.16 but can happen with a lower BAC if alcohol interacts with medication in your system or if you're female.[3] The BAC depends on your body weight and other factors when seeing how alcohol is metabolized by your system. For example, a 160lb woman who has five alcoholic drinks an hour would have a potential BAC of 0.16%.[4]

In severe cases, this can manifest as hours in which memories do not form and cannot be recovered. If you're lucky, you've never experienced the terror of waking up and realising that you have zero recollection of what you said, did or experienced throughout an evening.

I was more prone to passing out than blacking out, but a friend once described the experience to me. The last thing she could recall was doing shots with her housemate at a bar. She woke up the following morning, half-dressed in a strange bed, with no idea where she was, how she got there or who had been involved. Whoever's place it was, they were nowhere to be seen, so my friend hurriedly dressed and slipped out the front door. She was missing her handbag, but she recognised the suburb she was in and walked the 20 or so minutes to her home, where her housemate let her in as she no longer had her keys. According to her housemate, she had left the bar seemingly of her own recognisance. She had been dancing with a young man and appeared relatively lucid and like she was having a great time, so her housemate hadn't had any cause for concern. My friend was disturbed by this incident for years, struggling to reconcile the idea that she was somehow conscious, moving around, making decisions and talking but remembered none of it. It was her personal wake-up call to get sober.

And just to be clear - blacking out and losing your mind is NOT normal. If someone gave you a pill that would make you forget patches of the evening and put you in dangerous situations with men you barely know - would you take it?

4. ALCOHOL MESSES WITH YOUR PREFRONTAL CORTEX

The prefrontal cortex is the area of our brains responsible for planning, decision-making, and controlling our impulses. Alcohol consumption inhibits prefrontal cortex activity, leading to, funnily enough, your total lack of inhibition when under the influence!

What follows is the carnival of impulsive, rash, and downright stupid behaviour that can ensue when you drink a lot of booze.

Our memory and learning capabilities are also closely linked to the prefrontal cortex. This explains why we have such difficulty absorbing new information (ever had a drunk person ask you the same question over and over?) and remembering essential details (such as where we live or where we put our phone down while taking a piss).

Long-term alcohol abuse can lead to structural changes in the prefrontal cortex, significantly impairing the area's overall functioning. The consequence of this can be permanent and life-altering cognitive and behavioural issues.[5]

5. LOWERED INHIBITIONS = WORST JUDGMENT EVER

As alcohol decreases prefrontal cortex activity, our inhibitions start flying out the door. Sometimes, these lowered inhibitions lead to very funny stories. I can't deny that. There have been quotes that originated during nights out that my friends and I still laugh about to this day. But for every enjoyable memory, there are about twenty which make me full-body cringe at the recollection (some are still burnt into the back of my retinas as you will find out later, aka Karen).

For instance, my decreased prefrontal cortex activity led to me crying in the arms of the housemate of some guy who'd just rejected me (and so wasn't worth it). It led to the housemate practically having to carry my heaving and sobbing body home while reassuring me that the guy hadn't seen me crying over him (oh, he had). My decreased prefrontal cortex activity led me to pass out on the toilet floor at a wedding reception and start a fight with my date (my first time meeting most of his friends) when he tried to get me off the filthy tiles. My decreased prefrontal cortex activity led to me trying to sweet-talk my way out of paying a taxi fare (I was always broke) and the furious driver locking the doors and driving me to the police station while I sobbed in the backseat. Is that kidnapping? Probably, but I was in no state to invoke my rights.

The point is that very little good can come out of blatantly disrupting the essential functions of your brain in the name of a 'fun time.' Our bodies and our incredible brains have explicitly evolved to protect and help us. Having control of our words and actions and maintaining a healthy sense of inhibition is essential to getting along in human society and to self-preservation. Disrupting the brain region that controls your ability to make decisions, moderate your behaviour and control what you say and do is the quickest way to ensure you wake up with regret and maybe a lot worse.

6. UP WITH BOOZE! UP WITH BLOOD PRESSURE!

Saying that I was ambivalent about my physical health during my drinking days isn't doing it justice. I sincerely did not give a fuck. Now that I'm in my mid-thirties, oh, how things have changed. I cannot believe the things I used to casually put into my body, in more ways than one. I feel fortunate to have my brain's essential function working (*knocks on head*). Still, I have my share of issues that have to be monitored and managed. It's hard to know which of these was exacerbated by my binge drinking or how my past consumption may come back to haunt me in the form of future health problems, but it's comforting to know that I have potentially saved myself from worse outcomes by quitting when I did.

Let's talk about that health biggie: high blood pressure.

Alcohol consumption impacts blood pressure and can affect you in both the short and long term. In the short term, a night of binge drinking can cause an *immediate* increase in blood pressure. In the long-term, alcohol can lead to chronic high blood pressure, known as hypertension.

It is worth reiterating here that binge drinking, in medical terms, is considered to be 'four or more drinks within two hours for women and five or more drinks within two hours for men.[16]

High blood pressure is a significant risk factor for stroke, heart disease, and various other health problems. In addition, excessive, ongoing alcohol consumption leads to consistently poor food choices and the tendency towards a lack of exercise. Obesity is also a significant risk factor for high blood pressure.

A vicious cycle can occur when a person with high blood pressure is prescribed medication but continues to drink alcohol. Drinking alcohol while on blood pressure medication can increase a person's risk of fainting, becoming dizzy, and harming themselves in the process.

High blood pressure is a common condition that leads to various health issues. Uncontrolled high blood pressure, also known as hypertension, significantly increases your risk of:

- Heart attack/failure
- Stroke
- Aneurysm
- Kidney problems
- Vision loss caused by damaged blood vessels in the eyes
- Metabolic syndrome
- Changes in memory or understanding
- Dementia[7]

There are many ways to keep your blood pressure at a healthy level, including upping the amount of aerobic exercise you do, decreasing your salt intake, drinking more water, and reducing stress, but cutting out alcohol and quitting smoking remain the two top recommendations.

If in doubt, get it checked out with your Doctor. Poor health is a great reason to stop drinking and to get on that health kick you have threatened to do for the last few years (or maybe decades).

7. ALCOHOL IS A VERY, VERY WELL-KNOWN CARCINOGEN

Even though it's been decades since the World Health Organisation deemed alcohol a Class One Carcinogen, the alcohol industry has not been, let's say, *entirely forthcoming* in adequately conveying this to the public. And yet, if you check out the lists published by International Agency for Research on Cancer and the National Toxicology Program[8], there it is, somewhere between Acid Mists and Arsenic. Delicious!

To be clear, this is a list of KNOWN carcinogens. Not Probable, Not Reasonably Anticipated, not Rumoured-To-Be Carcinogens. Alcohol's link to cancer is *firmly* established.

The big alcohol companies have fought hard to keep any mention of carcinogens off their product packaging.[9]

Most liquor bottles and cans only carry a warning about the effects of drinking on pregnant women and the intentionally vague statement 'Alcohol may cause health risks'. I mean, no shit, my dudes. Sneezing while bending down to pick the remote control up off the floor may cause health risks (I once pulled a muscle in my lower back this way.) A tentative, shrugging "I dunno, alcohol may cause health risks, we guess" feels slightly different from a label explicitly stating that alcohol is a LEVEL ONE CARCINOGEN.

Because they won't tell you, I will. Alcohol increases your risk for the following cancers:

- Mouth and throat.

- Voice box (larynx).

- Oesophagus.

- Colon and rectum.

- Liver.

- Breast[10]

The body metabolises the ethanol in alcoholic drinks into acetaldehyde. Acetaldehyde can damage DNA, leading to tumour growth.

Alcohol leads to the impairment of the body's ability to break down and absorb various nutrients, a lack of which is associated with increased cancer risk. These include vitamins C, A, D, and E and carotenoids. It also increases blood levels of oestrogen, heightened rates of which are linked to the risk of breast cancer in women.[11] [12]

8. ALCOHOL WILL DESTROY YOUR BRAIN

Alcohol shrinks your brain. I don't know about you, but I find this thought profoundly disconcerting. Less shrunken brains than mine have broken the phenomenon down as follows:

The 'grey matter' in our cerebral cortex controls the brain's complex mental functions. The cortex contains neurons connected by fibres to different brain parts and other neurons inside the brain. These nerve fibres are the 'white matter'. The nerve fibres have many smaller threads called dendrites that reach out and allow the neurons to communicate with other neurons. The white matter and the dendrites are the most susceptible to the shrinkage that alcohol can cause.[13]

Strong evidence suggests that women are more vulnerable to the detrimental effects of alcohol on the brain. Alcohol affects women significantly more than men in a lot of ways. While studies have indicated that the brains of male and female alcoholics show similar levels of shrinkage and learning and memory problems, the difference was in the timeframe involved. The critical difference between the men and women involved in these studies was that the women claimed to have been drinking excessively for approximately *half* as long as the men in these studies. This is a strong indication that women's brains and other organs are more susceptible to alcohol-caused damage than men's.[14]

You might be thinking that women get a rough ride when it comes to alcohol (and like most other things in life!). For the most part, I agree, but when it comes to alcohol - take it as a sign NOT to drink rather than being disappointed we can't keep up with men!

9. ALCOHOL WILL DECIMATE YOUR MEMORY

So, what does all this mean? Decreases in white matter extend to fibres within regions such as the fornix, where messages are sent out of the hippocampus. The hippocampus communicates with other brain regions to process memories and help you retain information.

A damaged hippocampus affects a person's short and long-term memory.

Another thing compounding long-term memory loss in heavy drinkers is that people who drink too much alcohol have increased incidences of thiamine deficiency. Thiamine is an essential micronutrient that cannot be made in the body. It's necessary for growth, development, cellular function, and converting food into energy. Alcohol abuse inflames the stomach lining and digestive tract, which can reduce the body's ability to absorb vitamins.[15]

Drinking heavily can also cause a person to miss out on getting enough thiamine. As we know, heavy drinking can also induce vomiting, which robs us not only of our dignity but keeps the stomach and intestines from absorbing essential nutrients.

Thiamine deficiency can lead to dementia—specifically, an irreversible type of dementia known as Wernicke-Kersokoff Syndrome.

10. WERNICKE'S ENCEPHALOPATHY

Wernicke-Kersokoff Syndrome, or WKS, is a debilitating combination of conditions that directly result from thiamine deficiency. WKS is comprised of two different illnesses. The first of which is called Wernicke's Encephalopathy.

A triad of conditions typically characterises Wernicke's Encephalopathy: abnormal eye movements, a loss of muscle coordination, and confusion. Other symptoms may include memory loss, seizures and hallucinations. However, a patient does not need all these symptoms to have the syndrome.[16]

The condition is considered a medical emergency and requires immediate treatment with a high dosage of thiamine supplementation. If treated promptly, it can be reversible. However, if treatment is not sought, the condition can progress to a stage known as Korsakoff's Psychosis, a severe and permanent form of brain damage.

Still want that drink?!

11. KORSAKOFF'S PSYCHOSIS

Around 80 to 90 per cent of patients diagnosed with Wernicke's Encephalopathy develop Korsakoff's psychosis, which is characterised by a range of symptoms, including severe memory loss, issues with concentration, memory and processing, confusion, disorientation, inability to retain newly learned information, and difficulty with problem-solving. Symptoms may eventually progress to vision problems, tremors and even coma. Sufferers of Korsakoff's Psychosis may also exhibit a behavioural tendency known as confabulation, which is when they invent stories to compensate for the gaps in their memory.

Side note: I've heard plenty of made-up stories from my friends over the years as I would remember everything before I passed out, while they only remember bits from blacking out! What they thought they did never matched the reality. Confabulation seemed to happen most weekends, and that was without having been diagnosed with psychosis.

Once Wernicke's Encephalopathy has progressed to Korsakoff's Psychosis, it is still treatable with high doses of thiamine supplementation, nutritional support, and immediate abstention from alcohol. However, the prognosis is far less optimistic. The memory and cognitive function may be too degraded to be recovered completely, and permanent damage may ensue. Early recognition of the onset of Wernicke's Encephalopathy is crucial to prevent this outcome.[17]

12. ALCOHOL CAN LEAD TO HEPATITIS

Alcohol does various terrible things to our liver. One of the most widely known of these grave conditions is alcoholic hepatitis.

There is a common misconception that alcoholic hepatitis only occurs in cases of severe alcoholics. In actuality, it has been found that the disease can also develop in people who only drink moderately—especially if they are women. Women's bodies have more difficulty processing alcohol. It's why we get drunker faster, and it takes a lot less. Are you noticing we may get the short end of the stick when it comes to the effects of drinking alcohol?

When we consume alcohol, our livers break it down into acetaldehyde, a toxic substance. In time, acetaldehyde builds up, causing damage and inflammation within the liver. Inflammation within the liver can also trigger an immune response, resulting in scar tissue formation. This is known as alcoholic liver disease, which can progress to hepatitis, a life-threatening liver inflammation. Hepatitis decreases liver function, with the most visible consequence being jaundice which affects the skin and the whites of the eyes, as well as fatigue, abdominal pain, fever, loss of appetite, behavioural changes and even the eventual progression to liver failure or cancer.[18]

13. ALCOHOL CAN LEAD DIRECTLY TO LIVER CIRRHOSIS

Cirrhosis is severe liver scarring and can result from other liver diseases or chronic alcoholism. Cirrhosis develops in 10–20% of individuals who drink heavily for a decade or more. It is worth noting that a female 'heavy drinker' is defined as just eight or more drinks per week for women. Not per night, per week. I'm sure I'm not alone in being shocked by that definition, and it's unnerving to think how cavalier I was about teetering so close to severe organ damage.

As we've covered, alcohol causes injury to the liver through the liver by forming acetaldehyde, that troublesome compound which blocks the normal metabolism of fats, carbohydrates and proteins. Scar tissue is created in response to this inflammation, which makes it difficult for the liver to perform its vital functions, namely filtering waste products and toxins from the blood.[19]

Alcohol and liver damage is probably the most associated problem with drinking - but hopefully, the other 99 reasons in this book will open your eyes to how shitty alcohol really is.

14. ALCOHOL CONTRIBUTES TO FATTY LIVER DISEASE

Although it may sound more like a playground insult, Fatty Liver Disease is severe. In a literal sense, it's extra fat built up inside your liver cells, which makes it harder for these cells to do their job.

Here's where that pain-in-our-ass (or abdomen) chemical acetaldehyde reappears. A buildup of acetaldehyde and the inflammation this causes can disrupt liver metabolism, leading to fat accumulation in the liver cells.

A liver that is impaired in this way also has a decreased ability to perform the vital function of removing fat from the bloodstream.

As is relatively standard, women are at a higher risk of developing Alcoholic Fatty Liver Disease (AFLD). AFLD is considered a 'silent disease', as it presents few or no symptoms despite leading to a myriad of complications if unchecked, including an enlarged liver, hepatitis, cirrhosis, and liver failure.

Thankfully, AFLD is one of the few alcohol-induced health conditions that can be reversed once an individual quits drinking. Regular exercise can also make a difference.[20]

15. ALCOHOL WILL BREAK YOUR HEART

Alcohol does terrible things to your heart, and we don't just mean the way that your heart breaks when you drunk-order pizza but pass out waiting for the delivery guy, then jolt awake at 4 am realising that you missed out on your pizza. It does awful things to your physical heart too.

Alcoholic cardiomyopathy is the stretching and drooping of the heart muscle that occurs after long-term drinking has weakened it. This affects the heart's ability to pump blood, which is vital for nearly all of the body's primary functions.

Alcohol cardiomyopathy typically occurs in heavy drinkers who have a history of alcohol abuse between 5-15 years in duration. Heavy drinking is alcohol consumption that exceeds the recommended daily limits. This is under the guidelines of heavy drinking being more than fourteen drinks per week for men and more than eight drinks per week for women.[21]

One of the scariest things about alcoholic cardiomyopathy is that it rarely causes symptoms. Often, when symptoms do appear, they are those of congestive heart failure. These can include:

- Shortness of breath
- Fainting
- Fatigue
- Irregular pulse
- Loss of appetite

- Swelling of the limbs

- Concentration and focus problems

- A cough that produces frothy, pink mucus[22]

16. ALCOHOL INCREASES YOUR STROKE RISK EXPONENTIALLY

Alcohol increases the conditions favorable to stroke. As we've established, binge drinking leads to temporary and long-term blood pressure increases. High blood pressure is the most severe risk factor for stroke; the disease is linked to around half of all strokes in the UK.

High cholesterol is another substantial risk factor for stroke. The food we consume when drunk and hungover is usually drenched in saturated fat, the worst thing for our low-density lipoprotein (LDL) levels. I discovered in the last couple of years that I have a genetic predisposition to elevated cholesterol, and damn, am I conscious of what I imbibe now. But back when I drank? I was a full-time human garbage disposal. I had youth on my side, but it pains me to think how much worse my health might be today if I hadn't quit drinking when I did.

Thankfully, I never became a smoker. I was laughed at every time I tried to take it up because I'm apparently a 'bum puffer', which I'm absolutely fine with today. Bum puffing for life! However, if you're one of those people who've mastered the art of cooly inhaling and not getting heckled out of the room, you'll know that drinking alcohol increases the chance of reaching for a cigarette. Even if you've already quit. And cigarettes, I don't need to tell you all the horrible things they lead to, stroke being one of them.

Alcohol abuse is also linked to atrial fibrillation, which is linked to an increased risk of stroke, as well as the myriad of heart issues outlined earlier.[23]

17. ALCOHOL LEADS TO PANCREATITIS

While alcohol's detrimental effect on the liver seems to be relatively common knowledge, the pancreas has been somewhat neglected in the conversation. Truth be told, I had no idea what the pancreas even did before I began this project, aside from my vague notion that it was very important. As it turns out, the pancreas is critical to endocrine function, producing hormones like insulin and glucagon, which are essential to regulating blood sugar levels. It also makes digestive enzymes that help break down the food in our small intestine.

According to a statement from American Addiction Centers, "Acute pancreatitis caused by drinking too much alcohol makes up 17%-25% of the world's cases and is the second most common cause after gallstones."[24]

Long-lasting pancreatitis is an excruciating condition which leads to a variety of complications, including:

- Elevated risk of pancreatic cancer

- Obstructions in the gastrointestinal tract leading to vomiting and nausea.

- Obstruction of the bile duct, leading to bile in the bloodstream and jaundice

- Pseudo-cysts, which are collections of leaked pancreatic fluids, and can lead to pain, fever, a swollen abdomen and vomiting.

18. ALCOHOL DEHYDRATES YOU

You know what it's like on a night out. There's a certain point where you 'break the seal', and from that moment on, you need to pee every few minutes. And, of course, women's bathrooms always seem to have a line out the door and down the street...meanwhile, you watch guys casually stride into the men's room and out in seconds. We know dealing with the bathroom line is one of the many injustices specific to drinking as a woman. Alcohol is a hardcore diuretic, meaning consuming it causes you to lose more fluids and electrolytes than you take in.

In addition, alcohol also inhibits the production of a hormone called vasopressin, which is the antidiuretic hormone (ADH). ADH helps regulate the fluid balance of the body. The suppression of the ADH hormone not only makes you pee more but is the cause of the headaches and nausea you experience later.[25]

So yes, on a night out, you really are peeing much more than if you'd drunk the same amount in the form of water. Good times.

19. ALCOHOL MAKES YOU BLOATED

In my drinking days, I appreciated how beer was the one drink that could actually 'slow me down', mainly because, unlike a vodka and cranberry, or vodka coke, or a sugary cocktail, I didn't really like the taste of beer. Which made it the 'perfect' drink for those afternoons when I really wanted to have a nice time without the sesh turning into an event of some epic trauma. The problem was that beer bloated the hell out of me.

There's a reason for this. In the case of beer and champagne, you become bloated through the accumulation of bubbles in your stomach. As we've just covered, all alcoholic beverages have diuretic properties, and dehydration is another cause of bloating.

Alcohol also irritates the lining of the digestive tract in a major way, and this inflammation leads to bloating. The sugar and sodium content of various drinks is also a contributing factor to belly bulge.[26]

Then of course, there's the matter of alcohol leading to consumption of food that irritates the hell out of your digestive tract. Nobody drunkenly reaches for an apple. When I finally got my appetite back after a day spent moaning in bed with a ferocious hangover, the last thing I wanted to do was whip myself up a healthy bowl of oats and fruit packed with dietary fibre. My instinct was always to soothe myself after whatever abject humiliation I'd incurred the night before by snarfing down the greasiest takeout I could get my hands on—a surefire way to clog up my intestines for the better part of the following week. It was normal for me to have a stomach so distended and sore it'd be very easy to convince a stranger that I was going into labour.

Frequent abdominal discomfort is one of the things you may experience a lot less of when you finally give up alcohol.

REASONS 20-39

– MORE DEATH-DEFYING REASONS TO QUIT DRINKING (AND THE UGLY FACTS ABOUT ALCOHOL)

Let's just pause for a brief second to reflect on points 1-19 - what a shit show alcohol is for your health. You can't deny that alcohol is REALLY unhealthy in every shape and form.

Hopefully, your pre-conceptions of what you think alcohol is and the actual reality of it are starting to change. If not, here are another 81 attempts.

20. ALCOHOL SERIOUSLY AFFECTS YOUR GUT MICROBIOME, WHICH AFFECTS, WELL, EVERYTHING

The importance of gut health to your overall health and sense of well-being cannot be overstated. Yet, regular drinkers abuse their guts in a myriad of ways. For starters, alcohol alters the essential balance of bacteria in the gut, leading to a marked decrease in 'good' bacteria and a substantial increase in harmful bacteria. This can result in dysbiosis, a condition typified by the imbalance or disruption of the normal microbial communities in the gut. Symptoms of dysbiosis can include bloating, gas, constipation, diarrhoea, and abdominal pain. It has also been linked to various chronic diseases, including obesity, diabetes, and autoimmune disorders.[27]

Long-term alcohol consumption can also increase gut permeability, meaning it becomes easier for harmful bacteria and toxins to leak from the gut into the bloodstream.

Frequent alcohol consumption also impairs overall immune function, making it more challenging for the body to fight off bacteria and pathogens that may harm the gut.

Research has demonstrated that a healthy gut microbiome is essential to prevent the development of a range of chronic diseases, including obesity, autoimmune conditions, and diabetes.[28]

Gut health can even impact your mind! Poor gut health has been linked to the onset of depression and anxiety, which makes sense considering the discomfort and embarrassment associated with, well, having the shits a lot.

21. ALCOHOL MAKES YOU GAIN WEIGHT

One of the first things newly-sober people often notice is just how quickly and easily the pounds fall off their bodies (and those who don't, realize they have become addicted to food instead - especially sweets!).

Many people who consider themselves otherwise health and image-conscious; hitting the gym five times a week before work, counting calories during the day-seem to think that the calories they drink on the weekends somehow don't count.

Weight gain through alcohol consumption can be gradual and insidious. Alcohol itself contains seven calories per gram, and that's before you even start adding in the sugar and sodium content of your favorite beverages.

The calories in alcohol are empty calories. This means that while your body can convert the calories from your boozy night to energy, these calories contain few or no nutrients or minerals.[29]

Since your body works so hard to eliminate alcohol from your system immediately, it will prioritise this function. Your body will work to burn off the alcohol in your system before it burns off anything else, namely, all the carbs and fat you ingested while on a bender.

Not to mention the sheer sugar content of so many of the drinks marketed to women. Margaritas, daiquiris, and pina coladas, in all their enticing colours and fun and tropical promises, are usually jam-packed with added sugar and saturated fat.

I've known people who seem to be constantly on some restrictive diet, be it Keto, low-carb, no-carb, or intermittent fasting, who will take drastic measures to restrict what they put in their mouth when it comes to food, but wouldn't dream of cutting out their 'relaxing' evening wine or three. Alcohol effectively shuts down your normal metabolic function, yet it is often the last thing to go when people choose to overhaul their diets.

If you are stuck in a cycle of wanting to feel happier in front of the mirror, but trapped by being hungover and too paralysed to get your arse off the couch - stop drinking alcohol. It will help stop the cycle. The time and energy you will get back from not drinking alcohol will give you that time and energy you need to start making really awesome changes in your life.

Side note: These changes can involve getting yourself a super hot personal trainer as well.

22. ALCOHOL IS LINKED TO PSORIASIS

Alcohol usage can increase your susceptibility to psoriasis and can worsen your symptoms if you already have the condition. This painful autoimmune condition leads to thick, scaly and highly uncomfortable plaques on the skin. Even small amounts of alcohol consumption can:

- Make psoriasis worse or trigger a flare

- Disrupt the immune system, making it more challenging for the body to fight off inflammation and infections

- Decrease the likelihood of remission from psoriasis

- Make it more difficult for an individual to follow a treatment plan

- Interact with psoriasis medication, reducing its effectiveness

- Increase the chances of developing liver disease[30]

If you have ever suffered from this, as I have, you can understand how demoralizing it is for your own self-esteem looking like you have just been hit by a snow machine. If you want a potential remedy, never wear black and stop drinking!

Luckily for me, this was one of the first things to clear up when I stopped drinking, along with the next section (you are probably starting to build up a picture of me in my drinking days - and yes, it's not pretty).

23. ALCOHOL GIVES YOU ACNE

There has been some debate over whether or not alcohol consumption itself *causes* acne. Still, one thing is sure: it is a significant contributor to the conditions that can lead to the development and worsening of acne on the skin.

For instance, alcohol consumption can lead to bad habits like collapsing into your pillow face-down with a mug covered in make-up (guilty). Clogged pores are a contributor to the development of acne.

The effects of alcohol on the immune system also come into play here. Alcohol consumption can destroy the protective cells within the body that help you fight off infections. This may include bacteria like *Propionibacterium Acnes (P. acnes),* which causes cysts and abscesses.[31]

Alcohol consumption also triggers inflammation, which contributes to the development of acne by increasing the skin's sebum production. Sebum overproduction is also stimulated by the disruption of the body's hormonal balance, yet another thing that booze can contribute to.

This brings us back to the liver, which we discussed in detail earlier. When the liver is compromised and has an impaired ability to detoxify the body, this can also result in acne and other skin problems.

It's still a surprise to me, that I ever managed to get tv show appearances with the flaky, spotty and highly hungover vibes that I was giving off during my drinking days. Couple those with lowering self-esteem - it's hardly surprising that my alcohol intake increased as a result.

24. ALCOHOL MAKES YOUR BREATH STINK

Few things in life are as abjectly humiliating than realizing that you may be giving off some stink...especially if it comes from your mouth. We've all had the distinctly unpleasant experience of catching a whiff of somebody's 'booze breath' when they've had a few and started talking way too close. I shudder to think of how many conversations I had in my twenties that I punctuated with a sickly sweet cocktail or wine breath.

When you consume alcohol, it is primarily metabolised in the liver by enzymes. However, some of it is also metabolised by the bacteria in our mouths and throats. When these bacteria break down the booze, they release....get ready for it....acetaldehyde. Damn it! And being toxic, acetaldehyde smells like trash.

Then there is the diuretic effect of alcohol that we discussed in detail earlier. Dehydration can lead to a nasty case of dry mouth, and bad breath ensues when your mouth fails to produce enough saliva to wash away odour-causing food particles and bacteria.[32]

Bad breath can also be caused by lifestyle factors such as poor dental hygiene, gum problems and cavities. I'm going to tell on myself again; it's very hard for me to find the motivation to floss as a *sober* person. It goes without saying that I wasn't whipping out a ream of floss and giving my teeth a once-over before I passed out with a kebab or a stranger in my hand. As for regular dental cleanings, who could afford that? By God's grace, I am typing this today with all my original teeth. To everyone I breathed on between 2006 and 2016, I am aware and I'm trying to be better.

25. ALCOHOL ROTS YOUR TEETH

On the subject of how lazy drinking makes you when it comes to taking care of your mouth, alcohol consumption is a major contributing factor to tooth decay and loss. People who abuse alcohol long-term have increased plaque levels on their teeth and experience more tooth loss on the whole.

This is attributable to the high sugar content of certain mixed drinks, for instance, cocktails, and the high acidic content of certain alcoholic beverages like beer, wine and cider. Even low alcohol consumption affects your teeth in the form of staining. According to Dr John Grbic, director of oral biology and clinical research in dentistry at Columbia's College of Dental Medicine, "The colour in (alcoholic) beverages comes from chromogens." Chromogens adhere themselves to compromised tooth enamel, resulting in stained teeth.[33]

The dreaded dry mouth comes into play yet again since saliva helps neutralise the mouth's acids and wash away bacteria and food remnants. Without enough saliva, bacteria can flourish and cause decay.

If you're anything like me in my drinking years, there's the issue of how much you're exposing your teeth to stomach acid through the act of vomiting. It was part of the program for me to spend the day after a 'fun' night retching over the toilet bowl until I was dry-heaving because there was nothing left...effectively bathing my mouth in tooth-eroding stomach acid for days on end.

And if you suffer from acid reflux as a result of your boozing, where acid moves from your stomach into your throat and mouth (not sexy in any shape or form) that's even more acid chomping away at your teeth.

Giving up alcohol can save you from horrific (and expensive) dental surgery - because let's face it, nobody wants to go to the dentist if they can help it.

26. ALCOHOL MESSES WITH YOUR EYES

Our eyes give a lot away. They reveal our emotions through the way our pupils dilate and shrink. They are the gateway to our soul (and that gateway was permanently closed in my twenties). The small movements of our eyes can indicate whether we're lying. Crinkles around our eyes allow others to observe that our smiles are genuine. And our eyes make it pretty clear when we're drunk. That glazed, 'not all there' stare of someone in the throes of a bender is as disturbing as it is incriminating. No matter how 'together' you think you're coming across, the eyes can't lie.

Alcohol affects how our eyes perceive images (beer goggles, anyone?) by reducing the sharpness of our vision. It also slows down the reaction time of our pupils, making them less responsive to changes in our surroundings and in the light. This leads to blurry vision. The inability to focus on specific things is the cause of that 'looking right through you' appearance people's eyes take on when they're drunk.

So, if you thought you had gone home with Prince Charming after a heavy night of drinking and woke up to something completely different - that's your reason.

Alcohol also causes the eyes' blood vessels to expand, creating a bloodshot effect that can last for days. In addition, long-term alcohol abuse can lead to decreased peripheral vision or reduced colour vision over time.[34]

27. ALCOHOL MAY BE THE REASON YOU'RE LOSING YOUR HAIR

Thinning hair? It may not be just due to genetic factors or age. Your hair is another physical trait negatively impacted by your alcohol consumption.

This is because alcohol can interfere with your body's ability to absorb essential nutrients, primarily because of the previously discussed impact of alcohol on your gut health. Healthy-looking hair and hair growth require adequate absorption of vitamin B12, folic acid, zinc, and iron.

The diuretic factor of alcohol comes into play here, yet again. Dehydration affects hair follicles by making them more prone to breakage.

As we discussed in the acne and psoriasis sections, alcohol also wreaks havoc on the hormones in your body, including testosterone and oestrogen. This hormonal imbalance can lead to hair loss in both men and women.

Not to mention, the hard-boozing lifestyle gets pretty chaotic. The cycle I used to be stuck in was one of going out to 'forget about my troubles'-getting hammered-fucking up my life somehow-waking up full of regret-trying to put the pieces of my life back together-going out again to 'forget about my troubles'. This kind of lifestyle is typified by constant instability. Friendship and relationship breakdowns, job loss, and living paycheque-to-paycheque are all extremely stressful circumstances. Chronic stress has been linked to a condition called telogen effluvium, which causes hair follicles to enter a 'resting' phase.[35]

This is why, if you're a long-haired person like me and you're going through a difficult time, or a heavy drinker, you might find yourself swiffering the equivalent of a small child's head of hair off the floor every day.

28. IF ALCOHOL HASN'T MADE YOU WET THE BED YET, IT PROBABLY WILL SOMEDAY

As you may recall, drinking alcohol suppresses antidiuretic hormone production, which means it's not an illusion; you really do need to pee a LOT more when you've been on the sauce. If you drink to excess, the suppression of ADH continues after you've fallen asleep or passed out, hence the mortifying consequence of adult bed-wetting.

Alcohol also irritates the detrusor muscle, signalling that you need to urinate. In your inebriated state, your addled brain may miss this signal and fail to wake you in time to get to the bathroom.[36]

Unlike the other effects of alcohol on this list, this one mainly injures your pride. But do you really want to risk waking up in a piss-soaked bed next to someone you fancy? Even if you live alone and don't care (I hope you care), washing sheets is a whole thing, isn't it? Once a year is enough!

Then, of course, there's the urge to pee when coupled with a sense of inhibition that has completely gone out the window. One example is that of Landon Grier, a US man accused of exposing himself and urinating in his seat on a flight from Seattle to Denver. A federal criminal complaint was filed against Grier, who could face up to 20 years in prison and up to a $250,000 fine if convicted. According to Grier's defence, he had consumed "three to four beers" and "a couple of shots" before boarding his flight. He also stated that he had taken an "over-the-counter pain reliever because he had body aches from working" and couldn't remember the incident.[37]

29. ALCOHOL MAY BE WHAT'S GIVING YOU HIVES

Even if you're prone to these itchy bumps, it may surprise you to learn of the little-known connection between the condition and alcohol consumption.

Alcohol consumption can cause the body to release histamine, the chemical which acts as a protectant from infection and injury.[38] There is also the potential for an allergic reaction to the ingredients in alcoholic beverages, namely sulfites, grains, hops and yeasts.

30. ALCOHOL GIVES YOU ULCERS

Alcohol can "irritate and erode the mucous lining of your stomach, (increasing) the amount of stomach acid produced." This acid can cause severe damage to the lining of the stomach, leading to a condition known as peptic ulcers. Alcohol consumption can also increase the risk of bacterial infections, such as Helicobacter pylori (H. pylori), which is a common cause of peptic ulcers.[39]

Peptic ulcers are an excruciatingly painful type of open sore that develops inside the lining of your stomach and the upper portion of your small intestine.

Aside from the most common symptom of burning pain, peptic ulcers also lead to:

- Vomiting or vomiting blood — which may appear red or black

- Dark blood in stools, or stools that are black or 'tarry'

- Trouble breathing

- Feeling faint

- Nausea or vomiting

- Unexplained weight loss

- Appetite changes

Continued alcohol consumption also slows down the healing process of existing ulcers.

31. ALCOHOL CONTRIBUTES TO YEAST INFECTIONS

You're itchy at just the thought of it, aren't you? If you haven't experienced a yeast infection or a case of Vaginal Candidiasis, as it is known in the medical community, consider yourself very lucky. Quit while you're ahead, give up the booze, and save yourself from:

- Vaginal irritation and itchiness

- A burning sensation, especially when one has intercourse or urinates

- Vaginal pain and soreness

- Vaginal rash

- Vaginal swelling and redness

- Vaginal discharge with a 'cottage cheese' appearance[40]

Do you really need more reason to stop drinking than the term "cottage cheese appearance"?

Alcohol alters the delicate pH balance of the vagina, creating an environment that is highly conducive to yeast growth. This balance can also be thrown out of whack by dehydration. Those dreaded diuretic effects again!

Wine, beer, whiskey, gin, and vodka are all packed with yeast, thanks to the foods used in their creation; potatoes, molasses, beets and grape skins.[41] In addition, many alcoholic drinks contain high amounts of added sugar, which can also trigger yeast overgrowth.

So not worth it.

32. ALCOHOL UPS YOUR RISK OF STDS

You may have already figured this out on your own, but alcohol consumption leads to increased risk-taking behaviour, which often takes the form of irresponsible sexual activity. Strapping on your beer goggles and rolling home with a stranger doesn't just lead to feelings of regret and low self-worth, but can have lifelong health consequences.

Here is the breakdown of how alcohol consumption messes with your sexual health. When drinking, you may experience the following:

- Increased sexual desire, coupled with impaired thinking which leads you to forgo usual contraceptive measures (Have you got condoms? can quickly turn into shit, I'm pregnant. All because of alcohol!)

- The urge to engage in riskier sexual acts, such as sex with multiple partners or anal sex, which can increase overall exposure to the bodily fluids that transmit STIs.

- Lack of discernment in choosing a sexual partner and lack of forethought, such as asking the potential partner about their sexual history.

- The impairing effects of alcohol also increase the likelihood of becoming a victim of sexual violence, which can result in an increased risk of STIs.[42]

Just one experience of going to the STD clinic, especially when you see past acquaintances in the waiting area (true story), should be enough to put you off drunken sexual exploits. Sober sex is healthier sex.

33. ALCOHOL LEADS TO TERRIBLE SLEEP

Being a central nervous system depressant, alcohol has sedative effects. Although it can induce relaxation and sleepiness, and is indeed commonly imbibed for these reasons, the quality of sleep it produces is inferior.

Even a low amount of alcohol (and by 'low', we mean **ONE DRINK OR LESS** for women) has been shown to degrade sleep quality by almost ten per cent. Research has shown that while those who drink alcohol right before bed may fall asleep faster, the overall quality of their sleep throughout the night is poor.[43] As their liver enzymes work to metabolise the alcohol during the night, they are more likely to experience sleep disruptions. Alcohol reduces the amount of time you spend in the rapid eye movement (REM) stage of sleep, which is crucial for restorative and deep sleep. The diuretic effects of alcohol are what lead you to suddenly wake up at 4 am after passing out, with the need to chug a litre of water.

Finally, alcohol makes you saw logs all night. If you've ever tried to sleep next to someone who has had a few, you'll be aware of how loud it can get in that forest.

34. ALCOHOL CAN MAKE IT HARDER FOR YOU TO CONCEIVE A CHILD

Often, couples trying to become pregnant fail to consider how their alcohol consumption affects their chances. Studies by the CDC in the United States have indicated that binge drinking has a negative impact on the, for lack of a technical term, 'baby-making functions' of both men AND women. For the male, alcohol consumption has the potential to:

- Lower the testosterone levels, and raise the oestrogen levels, which drastically reduce sperm production

- Shrink the testes

- Cause premature ejaculation or decreased ejaculation overall

- Alter the size and quality of healthy sperm[44]

On the other side, heavy drinking can mess with female fertility by:

- Interrupting the menstrual cycle and ovulation

- Changing the hormone levels

- Causing hyperprolactinemia, or high prolactin in the blood[45]

If both partners are drinkers, even if their consumption is only considered 'low to moderate', the chances of a couple experiencing difficulty conceiving increase substantially.

35. ALCOHOL CAN RUIN YOUR UNBORN CHILD'S LIFE

Fetal alcohol syndrome is a severe and life-altering condition resulting from a mother consuming alcohol during pregnancy. How fetal alcohol syndrome manifests can vary from child to child, but the most common physical symptoms include the following:

- Differentiating facial features, namely small eye openings, a short, upturned nose, a very thin upper lip, and a smooth philtrum

- Slow physical development in utero and after birth

- Difficulties with vision and hearing

- Unusually small head and brain size

- Heart defects

- Kidney issues

- Bone and joint abnormalities

The syndrome also encompasses brain and central nervous system problems, including:

- Impaired balance and coordination

- Intellectual disability, a propensity for learning problems and developmental issues

- Poor memory

- Issues with the attention span

- A lack of problem-solving ability

- Difficulty comprehending the consequences of their actions

- Poor judgment skills

- A tendency towards hyperactivity

- Rapid mood swings

- Issues fitting in socially

- Problems with adjusting to change

- A lack of self-control[16]

36. THE EARLIER YOU GIVE IT UP, THE MORE CHANCE YOUR BRAIN HAS OF RECOVERING

Remember earlier when I scared you by telling you what alcohol consumption does to your brain? Brain damage in varying degrees is a severe consequence of long-term, heavy alcohol consumption, with even mild-to-moderate consumption linked to cognitive decline, particularly regarding memory. However, a lot of this can be recovered.

The National Institute on Alcohol Abuse and Alcoholism reported, "Certain alcohol-related cognitive impairment is reversible with abstinence. Newly detoxified adult alcoholics often exhibit mild yet significant deficits in some cognitive abilities, especially problem-solving, short-term memory, and visuospatial abilities. By remaining abstinent, however, the recovering alcoholic will continue to recover brain function for several months to 1 year with improvement in working memory, visuospatial functioning, and attention, accompanied by significant increases in brain volume, compared with treated alcoholics who have subsequently relapsed to drinking."

It also states: "Reversibility of alcohol-related cognitive function also may be the result of a reorganisation of key brain-cell networks."[47]

I am grateful every day that I gave it up when I did. I barely remember my twenties and had more near-death experiences than during any other stage of my life (mainly alcohol and high-heel-related). So it doesn't matter what age you are; you still have the rest of your days to fully embrace being sober.

37. NEUROPLASTICITY

Neuroplasticity is your brain's inherent ability to restructure or rewire itself when it recognises the need for adaptation. This typically happens in response to new experiences, learning and environmental factors. It is the process by which the brain continually reorganises itself, forming new neural connections and pathways and strengthening or weakening existing ones.

This ability to adapt is crucial to learning and development throughout our lifetimes. It enables us to recover after brain injury or trauma.

Historically, scientists and the medical profession believed that the brain stopped developing after childhood. However, research has since established that the brain is a dynamic organ which continues changing and adapting throughout our entire lives. Neuroplasticity is influenced by various factors, including genetics, age, experience, and environment.[48]

While this is promising, research also suggests that not all brain functions can be recovered equally.

While studied individuals who committed to abstaining showed improvement in the functions of short-term memory, long-term memory, and verbal fluency, the studies also indicated less improvement in the areas of visuospatial skills, semantic memory, sustained attention, impulsivity, emotional face recognition, or planning.[49]

Meaning that, even after sustained abstinence, and with the wonderful neuroplasticity of our brains, it may not be possible to fully recover all that we have lost. But don't be too discouraged. By taking action and quitting as soon as possible, you are giving yourself the best chance of returning to your pre-booze brain capacity.

38. ALCOHOL LEADS TO POOR SEXUAL PERFORMANCE

Alcohol causes a myriad of problems in the bedroom. One of the most well-known is that alcohol inhibits a man's ability to get and maintain an erection, or, in more graphic terms, 'Whiskey Dick' (have any male porn stars ever used that name?)

Alcohol causes Whiskey Dick and similarly affects the female anatomy (Vodka Vag?) by reducing blood flow to the area. Alcohol consumption also reduces sensitivity in the region overall, making it more difficult to actually enjoy sex.

As I said earlier, my two modes when I crossed over a certain drinking threshold were 'crying and grinding.' If I may be so modest (lazy) as to quote myself from the '101 Ways to Say I Don't Drink Alcohol' book' my standards when I drank dropped to the level of "any man who was remotely interested in me and even some who treated me with active disdain." For all our increased sexual interest, though, it's kind of a slap in the face that drunken sex is usually so, so bad.

Add into the mix impaired judgment via decreased prefrontal cortex activity, aka the thing that makes us jump back into bed with our ex who 'isn't really into condoms', and you have a lot of risk for very little reward!

39. YOUR IDEA OF 'NORMAL' ALCOHOL CONSUMPTION IS PROBABLY A PROBLEM (SORRY)

Signs and symptoms of alcohol use disorder are as follows:

- Being unable to limit the amount of alcohol you drink

- Spending a lot of time recovering from alcohol use

- Feeling an intense craving or urge to drink alcohol

- Failing to fulfil significant obligations at work, school, or home due to repeated alcohol use

- Continuing to drink alcohol even though you know it's causing physical, social, work, or relationship problems

- Giving up or reducing social and work activities and hobbies to use alcohol

- Developing a tolerance to alcohol, so you need more to feel its effect, or you have a reduced impact from the same amount[50]

If I'd read that list in my twenties, I might have been inclined to think, "But that's just what drinking is!" Who limits the amount they drink? The goal is to get shit-faced. Spending a lot of time recovering? A three-day hangover is just the price of a good night! Intense cravings for alcohol? Yeah, it's called '3 pm'. Failing to fulfil obligations? That's why I work a shitty job! If I get fired, I can get another shitty job tomorrow! Continuing to drink alcohol even though I know it's causing problems? What am I supposed to do? Raw-dog my social anxiety and feelings of chronic low self-worth? Not having hobbies? I'm not ten years old; going out is my hobby. Developing a tolerance? Admirable! Respectable! That's how you earn cool nicknames.

You see my point. What I took as a given were the signs of a severe problem. And this may be the case for you too.

REASONS 40-59

– THE 27 CLUB, ALCOHOL ISN'T HEALTHY AND STAYING STUCK IN A LIFE YOU HATE
(PLUS REASONS YOU WILL BE SHOCKED AT)

The bad health and death stuff will keep on coming as alcohol is a poison after all, so it's hardly surprising it's one of the main features of this book. We start venturing from the internal rotting and deadly nature of alcohol to more external reasons for giving up alcohol.

40. IT'S A LOT EASIER TO BINGE DRINK THAN YOU THINK

The Mayo Clinic identifies binge drinking as 'a pattern of drinking where a male has five or more drinks within two hours, or a female has at least four glasses within two hours.'

I was agog when I first learned these numbers. Four glasses within two hours? Do you guys mean 'my pregame'? My 'bare minimum to have a good night'? Yes, they do.

I've ruminated at length about why my own tendency to binge drink seemed to be so intrinsic from the moment I picked up my first drink, but there are other, more general reasons why binge drinking is just so damn easy.

Never underestimate the influence of peer pressure, no matter how old you are. In certain cultures that some of us grew up in that shall remain nameless (G'day), the *whole point* of drinking is to get 'p*ssed'. Or 'maggot'. Or my favorite, 'cunted'. It's just what you do to pass the time and have fun.

Also, in terms of drugs, alcohol is reasonably affordable. It's been a long time, but I generally 'survived' the lean times in my twenties with whatever bottle of piss water I could find for $5 or less. One bottle of cheap wine can go a long way when you're an underfed 22-year-old girl who drinks it really, really fast!

41. ALCOHOL MAKES YOU INJURE YOURSELF

Sure, alcohol-induced injury is funny when Luanne from 'The Real Housewives of New York' falls headfirst into a shrub. Or when Sonya from 'The Real Housewives of New York' falls off her chair at dinner and face-plants onto the floor. Man, the OG NY Housewives were the best.

More often, though, alcohol-induced injuries are serious.

Over 5.2 million people die worldwide each year due to alcohol-related injuries. Alcohol-related injury is the **third** leading cause of preventable death in the US. Alcohol-related injuries also account for 10-18% of emergency room visits, most of which are for head trauma. More of these victims are women, or middle-aged and older people, than ever before.[51]

However, the statistics may be even higher when you account for the fact that alcohol-induced deaths are likely under-reported. They may be classified under accidental injuries, traffic accidents, or falls, with the aspect of alcohol influence not necessarily noted on the death certificates.

42. ALCOHOL WITHDRAWAL IS ONE OF THE WORST THINGS THE HUMAN BODY CAN EXPERIENCE

If you have become physically dependent on alcohol, the process of detoxification carries with it a tremendous amount of risk. Over time, our bodies become used to functioning as best they can with the poison coursing through our systems. So much so that the act of quitting, especially cold turkey, can throw our physical systems into utter turmoil.

This section may seem counterproductive since my goal is to encourage you to stop drinking and stay sober.

This is why I'll reiterate again that, if you have any reason to believe you have a strong physical dependency on alcohol, you *must* consult with a medical professional before stopping your consumption completely. The earlier you do this, the better your chance of not experiencing the following symptoms:

- Status epilepticus, which refers to a type of prolonged seizure that lasts for 5 minutes or more or the occurrence of more than one seizure within 5 minutes. This carries a high risk of permanent brain damage or death[52]

- Stroke

- Heart attack

- Delirium tremens

- Burst oesophagal veins

- An array of complications due to electrolyte imbalances, including severe dehydration and anaemia[53]

43. THERE IS NO LEVEL OF ALCOHOL CONSUMPTION THAT ACTUALLY IMPROVES HEALTH

I think we've all heard the various rumours that, say, a modest amount of alcohol, like a glass of fine wine at dinner, can improve our health. Indeed, one of the most widespread of these ideas is red wine, in particular, is good for our hearts. The research behind these ideas has been indicated to be complex and contradictory.

In a blog for Johns Hopkins Medicine, the writer offers a hypothesis for why certain studies have shown a connection between a moderate level of alcohol consumption and a lower risk of heart disease: "It's hard to determine cause and effect from those studies. Perhaps people who sip red wine have higher incomes, which tend to be associated with more education and greater access to healthier foods. Similarly, red wine drinkers might be more likely to eat a heart-healthy diet." [54]

Conversely, excessive alcohol consumption is linked to a wide variety of health conditions that can lead to heart problems. I would argue that this effectively negates the slight and contentious possibility of any benefit. High blood pressure, stroke, cardiomyopathy, obesity and cancer are a few we have already covered.

44. DON'T TRY TO KEEP UP WITH THE BOYS: ALCOHOL IS HARDER ON WOMEN'S BODIES

The CDC has reported that alcohol use has 'unique health and safety risks for females.' The statistics are alarming for younger generations: a survey showed that about 32% of high school-aged females consumed alcohol, compared with 26% of males in high school. Binge drinking was also more prevalent amongst the girls than the boys surveyed.

'Biological differences in body structure and chemistry' are why women's bodies absorb more alcohol and take longer to metabolize it. After drinking the same amount, women generally have higher blood alcohol levels than men, with the impairing effects of alcohol taking hold more quickly and typically lasting a lot longer.

As such, women are acutely susceptible to the long-term effects of alcohol we've discussed previously. The risk of liver disease and cirrhosis is higher for women than men. Alcohol-induced cognitive decline and shrinkage of the brain develop more quickly for women than they do for men. Women have an elevated risk for heart damage at a lower level of consumption, and after fewer years of drinking, than men.[55]

Not to mention, it is women who are far likelier to become the victims of sexual violence as a consequence of excessive alcohol consumption.

45. ALCOHOL MAY INTERACT DANGEROUSLY WITH YOUR MEDICATION

Alcohol and prescription medication can be lethal, and far too many people are unaware of, or vastly underestimate, the risks involved in even having a few drinks while on meds.

Perhaps most commonly known is the relationship between alcohol and drugs considered central nervous system depressants, such as benzos and opioids. The combination of the two can trigger extreme drowsiness, leading to a heightened risk of falls and accidents and potentially fatal respiratory-system depression.

It is reported that 8.3 million adults in the U.K. alone take some form of antidepressant, with women twice as likely to be prescribed antidepressants than men.[56]

Influences like rising income inequality and the Covid-19 pandemic certainly contribute to the increase in depression and anxiety diagnoses, as does the increased awareness of mental health in general. For example, when I was a pre-internet pre-teen exhibiting my first signs of generalised anxiety disorder and OCD, there was no name for what I was experiencing, as far as I knew. I just thought there was something 'wrong' with me, that I was fundamentally flawed. I had no idea that anybody else in the world had 'intrusive thoughts' or tried to assuage these thoughts by enacting the 'strange' behaviours that I did. I firmly believe that an increased understanding of mental health is positive for society. Still, the connection between the medications prescribed to treat these conditions, and the negative interaction with alcohol, strikes me as under-discussed.

Alcohol can interfere with the effectiveness of selective serotonin reuptake inhibitors (SSRIs) and monoamine oxidase inhibitors (MAOIs) by reducing their ability to regulate neurotransmitters in the brain. This can actually worsen the symptoms the medication is intended to treat. You hear plenty of stories in sober communities of when people stopped drinking and a few months later, they were able to come off their medications as a result (always consult a Doctor first, though). I personally believe that alcohol can keep you depressed and until you experience the mental clarity that comes with three months or more of continued sobriety, the alcohol fog lifts and you start understanding how bad it was for your mental health.

Alcohol also lessens the effectiveness of blood thinners, leading to an elevated risk of bleeding and bruising.

While it seems most people know that they 'shouldn't' drink while actively taking antibiotics, I've seen more than one friend push the 'fuck it button' while on these meds and drank regardless. Drinking while taking antibiotics can get you very drunk, nauseous, and lead to serious illness.[57]

46. ALCOHOL IS ESPECIALLY DANGEROUS TO DIABETICS

People who experience diabetes already face various daily challenges when it comes to managing their health. If they choose to drink alcohol, their risk factor for all sorts of additional problems increases, namely the following:

- While moderate amounts of alcohol may cause blood sugar to rise, excess alcohol can actually decrease an individual's blood sugar level - sometimes causing it to drop into dangerous levels. This is especially true for individuals with Type 1 Diabetes

- The carbohydrate content in beer, sweet wine, and various other drinks may alter blood sugar levels

- Alcohol can stimulate appetite, causing an individual to overeat and mess with their blood sugar

- In a similar way, the manner in which alcohol affects judgment and willpower may cause a diabetic individual to make poor food choices

- Alcohol consumption and the poor food choices associated with it may also increase triglyceride levels

- Alcohol has a previously-discussed impact on blood pressure, which can lead to potentially lethal effects for people with diabeties[58]

47. ALCOHOL MAKES YOU RUN YOUR MOUTH

You've probably heard the quote "In Vino Veritas", which translates to "In wine, there is truth."

One of the misconceptions about alcohol is that it's a kind of honesty serum, that everything that comes out of your mouth is something you genuinely think and simply don't have the courage to express while sober.

This is a fallacy. Psychiatrist Omar Manejwala, medical director of the Hazelden addiction treatment center in Center City, Minnesota, said of drinking, "(You) may say things you don't mean and even things you don't believe." He added that heavily intoxicated people are also prone to telling entirely fabricated stories and repeating words and phrases they've heard before "without regard to their meaning."[59]

When alcohol is consumed, it affects the brain by increasing the activity of a neurotransmitter called gamma-aminobutyric acid (GABA), which has a sedative, calming effect on the nervous system. Alcohol also decreases the activity of the neurotransmitter glutamate, which is responsible for regulating cognitive function, and decision-making. As a consequence of these changes, the parts of the brain responsible for our judgment and decision-making become impaired.[60] Thus, our tendency to say whatever stupid shit pops into our heads.

Alcohol also affects our ability to understand and comprehend social cues, meaning we are not necessarily cognisant of how the stupid shit we're saying actually impacts the people around us. Someone in the throes of a drunken rant often seems to be on their own planet, with no comprehension or consideration for those around them and whether they're actually interested in listening to them yell about how lizard people are coming for us all.

I don't know about you, but in our current era, in which everyone carries at all times a recording device that can broadcast a video or live stream to potentially billions of people, I feel a lot better knowing I'm in complete control of every action I take and every word that comes out of my mouth!

48. ALCOHOL MESSES WITH YOUR MOOD

How I would describe my drinking days is, if I wasn't grinding, I was crying. I had three states under the influence: Convivial and Confident (this lasted 1-3 drinks), Inappropriately Flirtatious (drinks 3 to ?) And The Abyss. If my inappropriate flirtations hadn't secured me a companion for the evening, or if I had somehow been rejected, eventually the abyss was inevitable. The abyss was the buried, inner darkness that poured forth, all those years of trauma and suppressed emotion that would culminate in me sobbing in the bathroom, or on the floor, or in the street, or unleashing a fit of wild, out-of-character anger on the people around me. I thankfully never *physically* hurt anybody - but I have seen how bad alcohol and violence can be - you will meet Karen later. The abyss was everything I had been trying to avoid feeling. The abyss was the fear, shame, loneliness, embarrassment and a general sense of worthlessness that underpinned me for so many years.

It may feel as though alcohol is helping you to access 'the real you', but there is a purely chemical reason for all of this. Our bodies produce extra dopamine with the first few drinks. Dopamine, as you may be aware, is the famous feel-good chemical. We all love this shit and spend our days chasing it. Alcohol also cranks up the norepinephrine in the brain. This particular neurotransmitter acts as a stimulant. Elevated levels of norepinephrine increase arousal and excitement, lower inhibitions and increase impulsivity. This is how colleagues with no prior interest in one another end up in an R-rated grinding session on the dance floor. This is how the rollercoaster runs.

This is how you go from a friendly catch-up with a few friends to making out with your best friend, to being shoeless and shrieking at the bouncer that you'll see them in court. This is how a 'fun' night out ends in chaos which can cause another cringe-worthy half-memory (if you're lucky) or leave you dealing with the consequences for a long time if it's more serious.

Is it worth it?

49. ALCOHOL ROBS YOU OF YOUR TIME AND YOUTH

When we're young, it's easy to feel we have time to waste. We have our entire physical and mental capabilities. And we are myopic. It can be challenging for us to see the bigger picture, and to see past the desire for quick gratification and temporary excitement that is a boozy night out. It's all about immediacy.

When you feel as though you have time on your side, losing entire days to hangovers is fine. I sometimes went on benders that caused me to lose chunks of 3-4 days. And when I say lose, I mean that absolutely nothing was accomplished, apart from me lolling around in physical and mental turmoil. I often wonder what I could have done with that time. What if I hadn't spent so many days of my young life writhing in self-induced physical pain and crushing shame?

In your thirties, you begin to become shockingly aware of just how much time you've wasted. Where did those years go? The hours and days I spent hungover, lying in bed sick, my head throbbing, desperately trying to piece together the evening, mired in my shame and fear over something I said or did. What could I have used those days for, instead? How much could I have grown, as a person, had I not used alcohol to bury my sense of inadequacy and instead started confronting my issues years earlier?

While it is futile to dwell in a state of regret, we can use the past to inform the decisions we make in the future. With alcohol, history repeats itself.

50. ALCOHOL KEEPS YOU STUCK - SOBRIETY ALLOWS YOU TO HEAL

I've found myself, at times, suffering from a bizarre and self-defeating sense of "Well, I've already wasted so much of my life. What does it matter if I waste more? It's too late for me to do anything worthwhile. I pissed away all my youth and potential." This is ridiculous, and I wouldn't talk to my worst enemy this way. Yet, I often indulge in this thinking because it's a nice cop-out—a handy little way to feel justified in continuing to indulge in all my post-alcohol addictions and coping mechanisms.

For instance, although I've been sober from drinking for almost seven years, I'm much more recently sober from social media. I deleted my last holdout, my Instagram account, for good a few years ago now. My brain is still rewiring itself from that addiction. Without the infinite scroll of social media, I took to scrolling whatever nonsense internet content I could get my hands on. Worthless 'journalism' and articles from the trashiest celebrity tabloids. Obscure internet forums. Getting sucked into the Youtube algorithm for hours, only to be spit out the other side wondering how the hell I ended up watching so many 'Hair Fail' compilations. It's all just another way to never have to be alone with my own thoughts. Because when human beings are left alone with their own thoughts, the fear of their own mortality tends to arise. For me, this brings with it the sense that this life is all I have, and I'd better do something with it, but fucked if I know what. It's much easier to pick up the phone and scroll, turn on the TV, or pour yourself a drink. To siphon your mental energy into more and more miniature distractions instead of confronting the emptiness inside.

But that emptiness doesn't have to be scary. It can be a friend, and a guide, showing you what you really want out of life when you remove all the distractions and outside influences. How do you really want to be spending your time? You will be pleasantly surprised by what you discover when you allow yourself to sit quietly, take a walk, and just allow your inner voice to speak.

And if you don't like what those inner voices are telling you - upgrade your life with a therapist. My therapist was a complete game-changer for me. Having a place where you feel heard, safe and can work through the most traumatic parts of your past was one of the best acts of self-care I ever did.

And don't be one of those morons who say "therapy is expensive". Most cocktails in Los Angeles are $15 minimum these days. When you factor in other costs of a night out - you are probably looking at two decent therapy sessions. The level of self-growth you would achieve in those two therapy sessions versus a night out boozing, where you are continuing to sweep all those festering emotions of life under that bulging rug, are a world apart.

Don't be a moron.

51. ALCOHOL FUELS A SENSE OF LOW SELF-WORTH

Throughout my twenties, I experienced a deep lack of self-love, and I made the common mistake of thinking I could remedy this with romantic relationships. Asking a twenty-something-year-old guy to somehow fill the chasm left by a lack of maternal, unconditional love is a pretty tall order, and really not fair. In addition to this, I didn't really trust that I had much to offer, or that anyone could potentially love the 'real' me. And so I found myself, over and over, putting on the facade of the 'cool' girl who was totally fine with having casual sexual encounters, but still hoping the guys involved would want to make me their girlfriend.

I learned to substitute a man's sexual desire with a feeling of real affection, and that usually did the job for an evening or so. But whatever temporary feelings of self-confidence I had during the encounter were ripped away when the guy didn't return my texts in the days following, or made me feel like I was 'crazy' or 'needy' for expressing a desire to see him again (the horror!). I would sometimes see the guys I'd hooked up with getting into serious relationships, and it just served as confirmation that I was fundamentally unloveable. Please don't misinterpret me; I don't believe that there is *anything* wrong with having a F-buddy, or a one-night stand, as long as it isn't the consequence of you settling for something that is much less than what you actually want.

Heavy alcohol use is attractive to those of us who've fought lifelong struggles with low self-esteem, but it's also entirely counter-productive. Long-term alcohol abuse leads to a lowered sense of self-esteem in the long term. Our self-esteem is primarily affected by the following factors:

- Our own thoughts and mental concepts, including the ingrained beliefs we may hold about ourselves

- How other people react to, and treat us

- Experiences at home, school, work and in the community

- Illness, disability or injury

- Personality disorders

All of which can be negatively impacted, or highly exacerbated by alcohol use and it's after-effects.

And if you are anything like I used to be, I would worry about what people thought about me all day, every day. When I got drunk and passed out, I would then worry even more until I got drunk again. The cycle never stopped until I got sober and went to therapy.

52. ALCOHOL MAKES YOU LESS CREATIVE, NOT MORE

Multitudes of intelligent, creative people genuinely believe they cannot get in touch with their intuition or access their creativity without using drugs or alcohol. To them, it is integral to be inebriated to reach a higher plane of thinking and consciousness. It doesn't help that scores of immensely talented and creative people who've generated revered work publicly struggled with addiction.

It is all too easy to claim that drugs and alcohol are the elixirs that enable an individual to become their highest and most in-tune selves, to create art and write novels by obliterating their everyday concerns and helping them enter the free-flowing realm of the higher self. The addicted artist is a mystique, something of a legend. It's also a complete fantasy.

Successful artists/addicts are creative and brilliant not *because* of drugs and alcohol but despite drugs and alcohol. If the chemical element had been removed from members of the '27 Club' (explained in the next section), they would have been just as brilliant. And we would have had them for longer. Addiction and artistry often go hand in hand, but addiction must not be mistaken as the *cause* of artistry. There are many, many more addicts who never create anything, who squander their talent and their potential in the bar or deal with the chaotic aftermath of another squalid night out. For me, it was working a job I hated that exhausted me because I was trapped in the cycle of living for the weekend, with no time between the drudgery of my career and my boozing to actually take that writing class I had been thinking of.

There are many people who, when faced with the choice of whether to stay in an unfulfilling yet familiar life of living for the weekend, or to try something new, will choose to remain in the life they know and never explore the other possibilities of their existence.

Sobriety was the key to making life exciting seven days a week and not just for a couple of hours on a Friday night before I got utterly blotto (again).

53. ALCOHOL HAS TAKEN THESE TALENTED PEOPLE FROM THE WORLD

Growing up in my early twenties, we knew about the 27 Club and would joke about which one of our drinking friends was most likely to join it (pretty twisted looking back at it now).

Firstly, you don't want to be part of the 27 Club, especially if you are under 27 years old! It just happens that it's the age a lot of talented people have died from their addictions. If you have an ounce of talent, don't let alcohol ruin it. Here are some of the talented people who weren't so lucky (and slightly older than 27 but still too young!):

- Amy Winehouse: The English singer-songwriter was just 27 years old when she died from alcohol poisoning after a lengthy and public struggle with drug and alcohol abuse.

- Heath Ledger: The Australian actor died at 28 from an accidental overdose of prescription drugs, including painkillers, sleeping pills, and anti-anxiety medication. However, it was reported that alcohol was an additional contributing factor to his death.

- Avicii: The famous Swedish DJ and music producer was widely reported to be addicted to alcohol and painkillers to manage anxiety. He died at the age of 28 after he committed suicide whilst on holiday.

- Janis Joplin: The American singer-songwriter passed away at 27 from a heroin overdose, but it was also revealed that she had been consuming alcohol excessively, possibly weakening her immune system.

- Jimi Hendrix: The American guitarist and singer-songwriter also died at 27, with the cause determined to be asphyxia from choking on his own vomit.

- John Bonham: The English drummer from the band Led Zeppelin died at 32, also from asphyxia due to choking on his own vomit.

- Chris Farley: The American comedian and actor died at 33 due to a combination of drugs that included alcohol.

- Jim Morrison: The American singer-songwriter and poet died in the bathtub at just 27. Although no autopsy was performed, his demise was believed to have been caused by heart failure due to excessive alcohol consumption.[61]

As clubs go, it's a pretty shit one to join. Again, I'm grateful I made it to 29 and got sober. Whatever age you are, stopping alcohol can only be a good thing - if you're still not convinced - keep reading.

54. ALCOHOL CUTS YOU OFF FROM YOUR HIGHEST SELF

There is a misconception countless people have that they need alcohol to 'be themselves'. They assume that the artificially and chemically 'loosened-up' qualities they take on when drinking is who they really are. That it is the true self, the one that they're forced to suppress during the week, when work and family obligations take precedence over the free expression of their personality. They believe in 'earning' their weekends and the right to go out and be their most authentic selves. Drinking poison and losing control of their mental, physical and emotional faculties is their treat.

There is a way to experience being the most 'you' you have ever felt without alcohol. Without the potential of going too far and saying or doing something you regret. Seriously, if alcohol enables us to be our most authentic selves, why are these selves so often obnoxious and self-destructive? Is that you?

Whether we realize it consciously or not, most human beings, at our core, want to live what feels like a meaningful and purposeful life. But by settling for the temporary gratification of a night out on the sauce and enduring the dissatisfaction and disillusionment that comes in the aftermath, we distance ourselves from the possibility of attaining real contentment and lasting happiness.

55. ALCOHOL FUELLED-CHAOS ABSOLVES YOU OF HAVING TO DO ANYTHING MEANINGFUL WITH YOUR LIFE AND TALENTS

We've all known those people who seem to careen from one self-directed crisis to another. It's one thing to be going through a difficult time, but some people seem to make it their life's work to be constantly embroiled in some drama.

Maybe you're wincing because you suspect you might be this person. It's okay. I was this person all the way through my twenties. I didn't realize what I was doing then, but it's remarkable how quiet and chill my life feels now that alcohol isn't involved. Alcohol fuels chaos (you only need to watch Love Island to realize that!).

If I was drunkenly hooking up with a guy who treated me like crap, and then having meltdowns over his rejection, I could blame him for my misery. I didn't have to look deeper. If I got fired because I was hungover or late for work too many times, I had to scramble to find a way to pay my rent. Another life-consuming drama. If I tossed my glass of wine on a friend because I thought she was flirting with one of my previous ill-fated hookups, the ensuing fallout could keep me busy for weeks.

Conveniently, this left me with very little time to pursue the things that I claimed to want with my life. I had wanted to be an actor, but by showing up to auditions unprepared, hungover or even still drunk, I was protecting my ego. If I was fucked up, I could blame that for why I blew the audition. It protected my fragile sense of self from how I would feel if I actually tried my best and wasn't successful. It gave me an out.

Sobriety takes away the 'band-aid', and you are left with your raw emotions and the fact that you might be completely miserable.

Remember that therapist is only one phone call away.

56. ALCOHOL COMPANIES ARE NOT YOUR FRIENDS

Reclaiming your mind is the key to true freedom. It will enable you to cease buying into the lie that life is about simply working to acquire wealth and status in order to 'earn' the leisure time in which you drink and drug yourself into unconsciousness. The alcohol industry thrives on us squandering our potential, time, and relationships. Despite the insidious marketing campaigns that depict alcohol as the elixir of fun, friendship and good times, the industry is not letting you in on the secret to being your best self. Your best self is already within you.

The ways in which alcohol companies attempt to make their products an indispensable part of your lifestyle are seemingly endless. This book will lay out the truths about alcohol, which strangely enough, are the opposite messages you are hearing from the alcohol industry!

57. ALCOHOL REALLY MESSES WITH YOUR SENSE OF EMOTIONAL REGULATION, AND YOU NEED THAT AS AN ADULT

Alcohol consumption leads to an inability to exert control over one's emotional state. As alcohol lowers our inhibitions, the self-protective barrier between our pure emotions and their expression to the world is completely dissolved. As a result, the most minor slight or throwaway comment can kick off an all-out brawl.

This is particularly true when you drink to suppress painful feelings or memories. Many people, including myself, got into the habit of drinking to alleviate our self-consciousness, lack of self-worth and social anxiety. The kicker was that once I hit a certain point of drunkenness, the floodgates would open, and all of what I'd been drinking to forget would come rushing forth. And few things are worse for social anxiety than waking up and remembering that you snotty-cried all over everyone at the party.

Alcohol can affect our limbic system, the part of the brain responsible for regulating and enabling us to control our emotions. It does this by interfering with our serotonin, dopamine and GABA, the neurotransmitters that regulate our happiness and anxiety levels.[62]

58. ALCOHOL SCREWS WITH YOUR DOPAMINE ON A LONG-TERM BASIS

You've probably heard a lot about dopamine. It's the 'feel good' hormone. The one we spend inordinate amounts of time, energy and money chasing. It evolved to give us something of a 'pat on the back' when we do something good for ourselves, for instance, eating or having sex.[63]

By increasing our overall level of arousal, dopamine creates reward-seeking feedback loops. When we take our first drink, our brains are instantly flooded with dopamine. This generates that wonderful 'buzz'-the sense of lightness and euphoria that washes over us with the first few drinks of the evening.

The trap that I, and so many others, fall into is chasing that buzz by continuing to drink. Repeated and excessive alcohol consumption can decrease dopamine receptor density in the brain, which can ultimately reduce the brain's sensitivity to dopamine over time. This can result in a reduced ability to experience pleasure long-term, upping your risk of developing depression and anxiety disorders. Studies have shown that the brains of people with alcohol use disorder have fewer dopamine receptors, which are the areas of the brain where dopamine binds and activates neurons. Having fewer of these receptors means that the brain becomes less responsive to dopamine. This leads to the individual 'chasing the high' that they used to experience from drinking and finding it increasingly difficult to attain as time goes by.[64]

59. ALCOHOL LEADS TO MORE ARGUMENTS IN YOUR RELATIONSHIPS

My husband doesn't have a problem with drinking. He is one of those irritating, unfathomable people who can 'stop at one or two'. In our eight-year-long relationship, I can probably count the number of times I've seen him visibly drunk on one hand. We started dating a year before I quit drinking. And for that year, I'd say that our relationship was a little volatile. And it was mostly my fault. I'm not saying this because he explicitly blamed me, but rather because the self-reflection that has come with seven years of sobriety has shown me this truth. We almost never fight since I gave it up.

The arguments we had when I drank were so irrelevant and asinine, it was embarrassing. For instance, a few months into dating, we were at a bar with some friends of his that I'd only just met. He began telling a story about something that had happened YEARS before he even met me. As part of the story, in order to set the scene, he referenced an attractive woman who had been there. Him referring to another woman as attractive, even one he'd met years before he met me, activated my drunken neurosis so much that after he finished telling the story, I took him aside to chastise him in a hot whisper. "Why did you have to say the woman was 'beautiful'?"

"What?"

"You didn't have to say it like ', Then this beautiful woman came in'. Why did you have to say she was beautiful?"

"Uh...."

And on it went for the entirety of the evening. If you've had a drunken, irrational tiff like this, you know how it is. One of your insecurities gets activated, you're kicked off into a heightened state, and all of a sudden, you're arguing with your boyfriend in front of his friends over his inclusion of a detail in a story that took place *years before you met,* while his friends awkwardly sip their beers and try to pretend they're not concerned about the manic he's become involved with.

Even moderate drinking can lead a person to become 'more aggressive, disinhibited, defensive, sensitive, and irrational.'[65]

REASONS 60-79

– DON'T BE A KAREN (IF YOU WANT A FUTURE WORTH LIVING)

Don't be a 'Karen' (her real name has been changed for my own personal safety).

60. ALCOHOL ABUSE CAN MAKE YOUR PARTNER FEEL MORE LIKE A CARETAKER

Presumably, your partner wants to be with you because they desire a companion, not somebody they have to babysit. I've been on both sides of this equation, and neither is pleasant.

I couldn't tell you how many nights out I had like the one above, in which I started a tiff over some tiny slight or perceived indiscretion, forcing the people around me to spend the evening trying to console and placate me instead of enjoying themselves. I pulled this shit at weddings, birthday dinners, and other people's family events. I had the capacity to make an evening which was very much not about me totally about me, and my fragile, easily wounded ego.

On the flip side, I've also experienced playing caretaker to a heavy drinker. For a period, I dated a guy whose binge drinking eclipsed mine. He was in the hard-working/hard-partying world of finance, but unlike almost all of his co-workers, he wasn't into cocaine. Instead, he attempted to 'keep up' with the coked-up boys by just drinking more alcohol, which is as stupid as it sounds. He was a man who frequently called me so hammered he didn't know where he was, who often failed to even charge his phone. I couldn't fall asleep until I heard him stumble in at 3-4 am, and it was a constant source of arguments and tension within our relationship. He was a great guy when he was sober; generous, good-natured, kind and loving. But the resentment of all those sleepless, worried nights fractured and threatened our bond constantly, and ultimately it marked the first time someone else's drinking drove me away.

61. ALCOHOL CAN INCREASE THE CHANCES OF INFIDELITY

That pesky decreased prefrontal cortex activity again. It is often the case that cheating is the symptom of unaddressed issues and dissatisfaction within a relationship; however, alcohol facilitates the process by removing rationality and impulse-control from the equation.

Decimate the prefrontal cortex functioning, and suddenly it doesn't seem like *that* big of a deal for your marriage if you're sharing a little tongue with your work crush.

This impairment of the part of your mind that considers consequences is one of alcohol's most detrimental effects across the board. A decision that you make in a moment of impairment can irrevocably alter the fate of your relationship. It can create an erosion of trust that takes years to rebuild, if it can be rebuilt at all.

Then, of course, there's the previously discussed issue of the alcoholic blackout (not to be confused with passing out/falling unconscious), the condition in which you may continue to function more or less normally, while your mind fails to cement and solidify new memories. You can find yourself the next day with hours of time basically unaccounted for, a particularly distressing condition for anybody, let alone someone in a committed relationship.

62. ALCOHOL WILL HURT YOUR FAMILY

Excessive alcohol consumption doesn't just hurt your body. If you have a partner, children, or anybody you care about (this includes friends and chosen family), rampant alcohol use will take a toll on them in one way or another.

The examples of this are numerous, but for our purposes, we'll focus on how alcohol abuse affects the most vulnerable people in any family unit; the children.

Children who grow up in a household where one or more parents or caregivers abuse alcohol become captives of the unpredictable, unreliable behaviour of the alcohol user. They may witness domestic violence and arguments between the parents. They are far more likely to experience physical, verbal and sexual abuse than children who do not grow up with an alcoholic caregiver. They may also be forced to grow up too fast and become a kind of caregiver to their parent.

Even if the alcohol-abusing parent is loving and tries their best, children in this situation inevitably feel somewhat robbed of a childhood. My primary caregiver, my mother, didn't drink. Still, she had unchecked issues with her mental health that led to a volatile, chaotic environment at home. My high school best friend, on the other hand, had a loving mother, but one who struggled terribly with alcoholism. Although our mothers had different conditions, my friend and I have shared the same problems in our adult lives; chronic anxiety caused by a childhood spent in 'fight or flight' mode, a sense that we are not living up to our full potential, and the feeling that far too much of our youth was spent attempting to manage the issues of the adults around us. We didn't have the language for it growing up, but we knew that we were connected based on the sense that things weren't right for either of us at home.

63. DRINKING BUDDIES ARE FALSE FRIENDS

Alcohol consumption precludes genuine human connection. It may feel like you're nurturing deep emotional bonds when you're eyeball-to-eyeball with someone at the bar, taking turns to pour your heart out. But how meaningful can a conversation be if there's a good chance you or the other people involved won't even remember it? How often have you kicked yourself in the aftermath of one such drunken blathering session because you said too much, revealed too much, or worse, can't remember what you said or who you said it in front of?

When you get sober, some friendships inevitably fall away. You will realize that some of the people you considered good mates were only good mates because of alcohol. You might be shocked to think you've never even spent time sober with them! You may choose to meet for a coffee instead of a cocktail and find the conversation stilted or realize you have little in common. In this case, a few things can happen: you'll develop a deeper and more meaningful connection in sobriety, or you'll realize the only thing you had bringing you together was booze, and the friendship will end.

As much of a downer as this can be, it will free you up to form new connections based on more than the artificial sense of conviviality and togetherness that alcohol creates. And that's worth it.

64. ALCOHOL ABUSE CAN LEAD TO LONELINESS

Loneliness is a significant issue among people who abuse alcohol. Problematic drinking can lead to social exclusion and isolation from friends. Personally, my twenties were typified by such fallouts, whether that was because I had drunkenly rolled home with a guy one of my friends was interested in (there's no 'girl code' in a horny drunken rampage), or I had channelled my inner Real Housewife and thrown a full glass of wine on a pal because I thought she was flirting with a guy I was interested in (I'm still sorry, Laura).

The shame after such incidents also led me to withdraw and to many dark days with the curtains pulled, composing apology texts that I usually wouldn't send anyway. Often, my shame prevented me from even reaching out to apologise to people I had upset. I figured I was too irrevocably awful to deserve forgiveness, so I didn't even bother. I just let those friendships die. The shame exacerbated my existing anxiety and depression, leading to further withdrawal.

Studies on the correlation between loneliness and alcohol abuse have shown that people with alcohol use disorders generally feel they have less of a support network than people with other health disorders.[66]

65. ADULT CHILDREN OF ALCOHOLICS FACE LIFE-LONG STRUGGLES

The alcohol abuse of a parental figure will inevitably follow a child into adulthood.

Adult children of alcoholics are often hampered by people-pleasing tendencies and a 'saviour complex'. They may recreate the dynamics of their parent-child relationship repeatedly in their romantic lives.

A saviour complex refers to the tendency of specific individuals to always try to 'save' people. Adult children of alcoholics may grow up believing that their purpose in life is to subjugate their needs and desires to help others, as they so often had to repress their wants and needs in order to take care of the alcoholic parent in childhood. They are prone to finding themselves burnt out from expending all of their energy to help others in order to prove their intrinsic worth. In relationships, they will often be drawn to troubled, vulnerable and addicted people. They may become obsessed or determined to 'find a solution' to their romantic partners' problems as compensation for their inability to 'fix' their alcoholic parent.

Their intentions are good, as they frequently believe they can turn their adverse childhood experiences into something positive in this way, but they often find themselves wounded and stuck in the same cycle, unable to truly induce change in their partner, feeling just as helpless and ineffectual as they did when they were a child. Adult children of alcoholics frequently find themselves experiencing depression and a sense of failure.

66. PARENTING WITH HANGOVERS IS TRULY NIGHTMARISH

If you're not yet a parent but are planning to become one, it's probably best you get a jump on the whole sobriety thing now so you never have to endure the hopeless despair of realizing you have an entire Saturday of kid commitments ahead while you're dealing with a brain-compressing headache, a dry mouth and an overwhelming sense of regret.

It might be hard to imagine when you're fully immersed in your own misery, but if you're hungover a lot, it can really impact your children. We understand that adult children of alcoholics deal with lifelong issues, but even if you aren't visibly hungover consistently, or you think you hide it well, you are far more likely to be short-tempered, irritable, snappy, uncommunicative and unenthusiastic about your parental duties and children's events when you're nursing a hangover.

Sometimes something that seems relatively innocuous to you will stick in your child's mind for a long time. A child will remember your lack of enthusiasm, how you appeared tired and bored at their football game, or instances when you snapped at them. You never know how the seemingly small consequences of your hangover could impact them and how they view you.

67. THE OFFICE CHRISMAS PARTY CAN RUIN YOUR LIFE

A survey carried out by afterdrink.com has indicated that *one in ten* people in Britain has faced disciplinary action or even been fired after getting too boozy at the office Christmas party.

In follow-up responses, 23% of survey participants who'd been fired after a Christmas party stated it was because they'd said something inappropriate, 21% said it was because they'd gotten into a verbal or physical fight with a colleague or boss, 16% said they'd been caught doing drugs, and 14% said it was because they'd been caught having sex with a colleague. A further 11% said they'd been reprimanded or let go for nudity or inappropriate comments.[67]

If you have ever forgotten what you did or said at an office party and had the dreaded work anxiety the following day, you know how terrifying it is that you could get fired for something you can't remember - don't let alcohol ruin your career for the sake of a few hours of mindless 'fun'.

68. ALCOHOL MAKES YOU PERFORM WORSE AT WORK, PERIOD

It's not always the prospect of your once-a-year humiliation at the Christmas party that you need to worry about. No matter how much faith you have in your ability to 'keep it together' whilst hungover (or still drunk) at work, your performance IS being affected.

Alcohol consumption and its after-effects impair concentration (having to focus on a spreadsheet with a throbbing head and bile rising in your throat is undoubtedly one of the circles of hell). You might think those days where you spend half the day half-dozing at your desk, and the other half on the toilet diddling your phone because you can't deal with work are just 'one day', but those days add up. If you do it enough, they add up to weeks, even months, even years, that you're not performing to the best of your abilities. If you are interested in progressing at your job and aren't just there to punch the clock, this is a problem. Your colleagues will notice. The people responsible for giving you a raise or promotion will notice. The people you'll need to provide you with a reference when you want to move on will notice. Sloppy work, missed deadlines and general half-arsery eventually gets noticed, no matter how much you hide in the bathroom.

As does absenteeism, especially if you broadcast your evening on social media and forget to 'mute' your co-workers and managers (rookie). They know you don't have Covid for the fifth time this year, and if you do, it's because you caught it from that dude you were grinding in the Insta story you posted at 4 am.

Then there are the potential legal issues. Driver Under the Influence (DUI) and public intoxication charges can be dire for your career prospects, especially if you work in an industry where background checks or security clearance is required for employment. This type of information is often readily available online to anybody who wishes to search you via the many and constantly multiplying data broker websites.

69. SOBER PEOPLE MAKE MORE MONEY

I'm not a fan of 'hustle culture', this pervasive 'rise and grind' mentality that reduces human beings to their constant productivity, usually in service of a system that doesn't really serve them all that well. So I won't scream at you to rise and grind and fill your days with constant action here, unless that's really how you like to roll. Personally, I'm more of a fan of 'Deep Work', the idea popularised by Cal Newport and expanded upon in his book of the same name. Deep Work is the opposite of the multi-tasking culture that's come to dominate. The culture that says you ought to be maximising every minute, running on the treadmill while listening to motivational podcasts while composing emails while live-streaming yourself to build your 'brand'. I don't think sobriety necessarily helps your career because it enables you to fill your hangover-free time with back-to-back activities (again, unless you like being busy), but rather, because it allows you to concentrate intensely on one thing. Deep concentration is the key to true mastery. The focus you regain from not being hungover will enable you to achieve this state.

Imagine sitting at your desk on Monday morning and being ready to tackle what's in front of you rather than being sick to your stomach, hungover, and full of dread? Then imagine being consistently productive at what you do - without those days where you are literally pushing paper around your desk and taking an obscene amount of toilet and coffee breaks hoping that clock will magically strike 6 pm. When you remove the effects of alcohol from your career - positive things start happening fast.

And if you have a job you'd love to get the hell out of, even better. When you get off work, instead of heading straight to the bar or going home to finally collapse from your hangover, you may find yourself with the motivation to work on your own business idea, the thing that really gets you excited. Or to take a course that enables you to learn new skills in service of a career path you may prefer. Or do some cheeky job-hunting and resume-tweaking. You can begin to formulate an exit strategy. Sobriety gives you back power and agency in this way. When your off-work hours are totally yours, you can start to reclaim your time and life.

70. THE COST OF A NIGHT OUT

If the massive hits dealt to your ego and sense of self-worth after a blow-out night on the town aren't enough reason to quit, how about some hard numbers?

I did the majority of my drinking while living in Sydney, Australia. In Sydney's Eastern suburbs and CBD area, a beer at a bar can set you back up to $12, with a glass of house wine at some Sydney spots ranging from $10-$13. Suppose you have a taste for fancy cocktails. In that case, you're looking at $20 a pop easily at most venues where you'd actually want to get a cocktail. So a mellow night involving just three drinks could be $60 down the toilet to barely get your buzz on. And it was never just three drinks. I mean, come on. Throw into the mix taxi or rideshare fare (let's say at least $30 late at night) and an entry fee of $10-$20 at whatever ridiculous sceney club my worst friends insisted on going to. What about take-away the next day when I was hungover? $30-40. Given that I could only hold down retail jobs, it's no wonder I usually just downed the cheapest bottle of wine I could get my hands on before I left the house.

And don't get me started on smoking! $25 dollars for a pack of 20 cigarettes in Sydney. Luckily I never got into smoking but my friends would always complain about the extortionate price of cigarettes.

The problem is - it's not just a night out. Imagine the money you could have saved for something else? That car, that house, that Mulberry handbag you always thought was out of your budget.

From the act of quitting drinking, I found myself with money left over each month, which I saved, and this was coupled with the fact that I was performing 100x better in my job and more money accumulated as a direct result.

This was the polar opposite of what an alcohol lifestyle was doing to my bank balance. I would get paid, drink it all away on 'fun' nights out that we barely remember (and if we did, it was highly confabulated) and end up in debt each month, driven mainly by a 'fear of missing out' (FOMO). More on that later.

If I wanted to go to the local Mulberry store next week to actually buy something (rather than pretending I could) - I can, and I have (a few times). All thanks to sobriety.

71. ALCOHOL IS A LIFESTYLE INVESTMENT THAT RETURNS NOTHING

If you think going on nights out and barely remembering what happened is a good investment of your time, energy and money - think again.

What do you have to show for with the money you spent on going out? A banging headache? More acne? A questionable man in your bed?

Alcohol as an investment produces negative equity - it robs you of all the money you spent, it makes you lazy for days after, it leaves you feeling depressed and stops you from investing your time in self-growth. You get NOTHING in return for an alcohol life-style that leaves you feeling empty inside.

Money talks - so in this example, we will use lots of it.

Just imagine for a moment that you stopped drinking back in the day when Crypto just took off. Yes, it could be argued now (or again at some other point when it inevitably rises sharply in value and crashes again) that you would have to be drunk to 'invest' in something so volatile. But hear me out.

If you were hungover most weekends and living pay-cheque to pay-cheque as I had, the want and need to invest in anything that might help you grow as a person (or as a filthy rich person in this case), would have felt like climbing Mount Everest in high heels. Ordering pizza and changing Netflix documentaries was hard enough.

That sober version of you is 100x more likely to see investment opportunities, whether monetary, relationship, emotional, self-growth or career-related investments.

So if you were sober when Crypto first launched, you might have had the time and energy to see the opportunity ahead (rather than binge-watching crime documentaries whilst covered in pizza and chocolate). If you invested $1000 at the time of launch and sold those shares at the highest share price eleven years later - you would now have just under $800,000,000.

Or more realistically, you could have invested in your favorite Mulberry handbag and five years later exchanged it for a newer design and actually made money on your original investment (true story).

While I have minimal attachment to material things (apart from my Mulberry handbags), my point is this - sobriety allows you to invest in areas of your life that can really grow exponentially compared to being hungover and unhappy when under alcohol's control.

72. DRUNK DRIVING KILLS, MAIMS AND DESTROYS

I first learned of Jacqueline 'Jacqui' Saburido when I was a teenager through an anti-drunk driving campaign which was circulated as a forwarded email. Her face and her story have hardly left my mind since. I never learned to drive, so I can, by default, say I never drove while under the influence. However, I think of

Jacqueline whenever someone I know casually mentions getting behind the wheel of a car when they've had too many. Truthfully, I think of her every time I get into a car, period.

Jacqui was 20 years old and had recently arrived in the US from her native Venezuela to study English. Jacqui was travelling home from a party with some friends when the car they were in was hit by an 18-year-old named Reginald Stephey, who had a blood alcohol level of 0.13 (0.08 was the limit at the time). While Reginald was unharmed, the collision killed the driver of Jacqui's car and another passenger. Two more passengers were pulled from the vehicle before it went up in flames.

Jacqui, however, was trapped. She reportedly burned for at least a minute before paramedics could extinguish the fire. She had third-degree burns to almost her entire body, including her face and scalp. She lost her lips, ears, eyelids, nose and fingers. In the years following the accident, she endured over 100 operations. Her devoted father, Amadeo, put his life on hold to give her the around-the-clock care she required until her death from cancer at 40 years old. Reginald Stephey's decision to drive drunk irrevocably condemned a young woman to a short life of physical and emotional anguish. It also destroyed the high-school football player's ambitions for his future. Reginald was released from prison nine years later.

Jacqueline and Reginald represent just two of the countless lives ruined by a split-second decision to drive under the influence.[68]

73. BINGE DRINKING LEADS TO AN INCREASED RISK OF HOMICIDE

Studies indicate a strong correlation between alcohol consumption and the heightened possibility of becoming either a victim or perpetrator of a homicide. Using data on 1,887 convicted homicide offenders, a study conducted by the Research Institute on Alcoholism in Buffalo, New York, demonstrated that about 50 per cent of the homicide perpetrators surveyed were under the influence of alcohol when they committed their crimes.

"A heavier style of drinking is much more prevalent among homicide offenders than in the general population", it was reported. "A direct role for alcohol is indicated by the finding that homicides were associated with a heavier than usual episode of drinking and the large mean alcohol consumption contiguous to the crime (9.3 ounces of alcohol or about 18 drinks)."[69]

74. BINGE DRINKING LEADS TO AN INCREASED RISK OF SUICIDE

The Substance Abuse and Mental Health Service Administration (SAMHSA) has established a link between alcohol misuse and suicide risk that is an unfathomable TEN TIMES greater than the general population.

Alcohol leads to decreased prefrontal cortex activity (the prefrontal cortex being the part of the brain responsible for decision-making, rationality and considering the consequences of one's actions). It can cause the user to plummet to excruciating mental lows. All of a sudden, a person dealing with some manner of emotional upset or trauma, or even the old wounds that can sometimes open back up when we've had a few too many, is stripped of their ability to think clearly, to see a way out, to utilise coping strategies they may use if they were sober.

Alcoholism often develops as a coping mechanism for an individual struggling with another mental health disorder. As a long-term anxiety sufferer due to my home life putting me in constant fight-or-flight mode, I drank to feel somewhat comfortable in the world. To alleviate the constant pulse sense of impending doom, the neurosis, the sense that something was always about to go horribly wrong, that underpinned my every sober moment. I'm not alone in this; many people experiencing mental illness or PTSD drink as a form of self-medication, to disastrous effect. The worst of these is the decision to end their lives. Alcohol can unearth things you didn't know you felt and expose psychological vulnerabilities you cannot deal with while under the influence.[70]

75. ALCOHOL REMOVES YOUR SEXUAL AGENCY

Alcohol robs you of your discernment in who you let into your bed. Speaking from my perspective as a woman, so many forces are conspiring to deprive us of our agency and autonomy. Advertisers and marketing executives labour to convince us that our faces and bodies aren't good enough, just as they are, in order to sell us snake-oil cosmetics and increasingly bizarre and dangerous procedures. Politicians and lawmakers use our bodies and the issue of reproductive choice as political battlegrounds. Being clear-headed about the people you allow into your physical space enables you to take some of your power back. Alcohol makes you see terrible prospects as reasonable and desirable. It removes your sense of choice from the matter rather explicitly.

As I said previously, I spent a great deal of time chasing after the sense of self-worth I lacked through casual sexual encounters. I played the part of the party girl who was totally cool with hooking up and never being called again, but I wasn't. Make no mistake, I don't think there's anything wrong with casual sex if you decide to partake of your own volition. But it wasn't what I wanted. I would just drink too much, and it happened. What I truly wanted was to be loved, but I really didn't believe or trust that anyone would be interested in me if I didn't offer them sex immediately. The momentary, fleeting high of a person's sexual attraction to me was a placeholder for love. It did its job for an evening, but I knew that long-term, it was only breaking me down.

76. ALCOHOL IS A REPUTATION KILLER

At this point, it may be worth consolidating how excessive alcohol consumption harms your personal and professional reputation and the long-term damage this can do to your life.

Individuals with a pattern of inappropriate behaviour, both in social and professional settings, face ostracisation and the impediment of their opportunities for professional growth. The ubiquity of social media means that such infractions now have the potential to reach a global audience. The offensive joke you told loudly at the Christmas party (complete with physical act-outs and character voices) is no longer just a matter of concern for the people who were actually there. It could go viral, affecting your prospects in every area of life, for the rest of your life. The internet is forever.

When I look back on my twenties, I still feel a lot of shame. It's difficult not to when you've repeatedly made decisions that go against your better judgment and nature. There are people I will never have the chance to apologize to. Even if I did apologize, I don't know if they'd be receptive to it, or if it would even matter. The damage was done. I'm not proud of who I was when I was drinking heavily, and that's something I will always have to live with. Regret is ultimately futile, and we cannot change the past. Taking control of the rest of your life is the only choice you have.

And if you decide to try out Alcoholics Anonymous meetings and do the 12 steps - you will get the chance to 'make amends' to those that you hurt (who are still around and it wouldn't make things worse). I can safely say this was the most terrifying and relieving experience of my life!

77. ALCOHOL IS A GATEWAY TO HARDER DRUGS

The gateway drug theory suggests that legal drugs like tobacco and alcohol can lead to the abuse of illicit, 'harder' drugs. You've almost certainly seen this theory in action on a night out or participated in the 'study' yourself. The lowered inhibitions and prefrontal cortex activity accompanying alcohol intoxication lead to a cascade of terrible decisions. Suddenly, doing a line with the wild-eyed guy who gave you the creeps at the beginning of the night doesn't seem like the bad idea it most definitely is.

'Party' drugs are more dangerous than ever. The Guardian reported, "The rate of cocaine-related deaths among women has increased by more than 800% in the last 10 years."[71]

78. ALCOHOL LEADS TO LIFE-CHANGING VIOLENCE (COWARD PUNCHES AND KAREN)

In 2014, New South Wales, Australia, introduced the law known as the "one-punch law". It resulted from community outrage over the deaths of two young men from single blows to the head incurred during separate nights out in Sydney. Offenders convicted of fatal one-punch assaults while under the influence of drugs or alcohol face minimum eight-year sentences in New South Wales.[72]

And before you start assuming this is largely targeted at men.....

My old drinking buddy Karen (not her real name) could be one hell of a bitch when she went past that illusive 'tipping point' from having memorable fun to being a bad cunt (FYI - Aussies categorize people as being either good cunts or bad cunts. Bad cunts are not something to aspire too!). It dawned on me that I may have been unconsciously drawn to drinking alongside her due to the comforting validation it gave me about my own habits. But despite her overtly flirtatious behavior and the negative "bad bitch" energy she projected, she always seemed to avoid any repercussions.

Until she didn't.

We were in the club, dancing on the dancefloor near some guys, and she said she felt a nudge from another girl behind her. No big deal; it always happens in clubs. Then it apparently happened again (still no big deal), and in under two seconds, she went from bad bitch to criminal bitch, and that was the last time I saw Karen.

Karen's sudden outburst of alcohol-fueled rage caused her to swing her arm at the woman she accused of nudging her. In the chaos, her glass of vodka cranberry went flying and shattered across the other girl's face, leaving her with a serious injury from being "glassed." It was a jarring scene, reminiscent of the type of violence usually associated with men who have suffered from years of neglect and unresolved anger management issues - not something you would expect from a 5-foot-6-inch, outspoken Australian woman who worked in finance.

Even now, the memory of the girl's face covered in a thick layer of blood, obscuring any discernible features and revealing a large gash across her eye - which ultimately robbed her of her vision - is seared into my mind's eye.

Karen got three years in jail for an action that took less than two seconds. All because of alcohol and probably a tonne of unresolved trauma in her life - which is likely to be another reason we bonded originally.

Moral of this story (and this book) - don't be a Karen! Get sober, go to therapy and don't let a senseless alcohol induced fit of rage ruin the rest of your life.

Even if you don't class yourself as a 'Karen', it only takes one incident where you have had too much to drink to alter the rest of your life.

79. ALCOHOL IS BAD FOR THE PLANET

While it's a positive step that so many people are becoming conscious of the environmental impact of things like the clothes they buy and the food they consume, what alcohol production does to our world has been little discussed.

On a basic level, we have a limited amount of land on which to grow food, and that viable land is growing more and more scarce. Food is essential to human life, and alcohol is not. But we are continuing to use vast amounts of our remaining viable land for its cultivation.

As reported in the Independent: "It is not just land that is scarce – water supply is at a premium in many regions across the globe. As global consumption of alcohol increases, so does the demand for water used to irrigate crops and manufacture alcohol. One 500ml bottle of beer uses 148 litres of water – and a single 125ml glass of wine, 110 litres."[73]

Most crops grown to produce alcohol are also doused with pesticides, contributing to the pollution of local waterways. In addition, the production, transportation, and distribution of alcohol results in significant greenhouse gas emissions.

REASONS 80-101

– THE MEANING OF LIFE, UN-BITCHING AND SOBER DATING (AND WHY SOBER SEX IS BETTER SEX)

If you haven't been convinced to stop drinking yet (or to stay sober), then God help you. But before you need an intervention, here are my last attempts to try and convince you.

80. ALCOHOL COULD GET YOU BANNED FROM FLYING

If you're newly sober or sober-curious, you might experience a moment of panic that takes the form of, "But how am I gonna cope when I fly?"

Many people feel as though they need alcohol to take the edge off when they travel, whether it be because they are nervous, easily irritated by being crammed into close quarters with often-inconsiderate strangers, bored, or wanting to pass the time by falling asleep. It's understandable. But it's incredibly ill-advised.

For starters, you are more likely to become intoxicated, at a faster rate, than on the ground. As Dr Karen Jubanyik, an associate professor of emergency medicine at Yale University School of Medicine, says, "There is usually very little food available on most flights — or it is not particularly appetising — and it would be easy to drink too much on a relatively empty stomach."[74]

As anyone with an internet connection is probably aware, 'drunk passenger removed from plane' is a headline that has become relatively common over the last few years. There was a time when being kicked off a flight for unruly behaviour may have been humiliating and costly, but it wouldn't have made international news. Those days are over, for better or worse.

The expression 'the crowdsourced panopticon' was coined by journalist and author Adam Greenfield in his book "Radical Technologies: The Design of Everyday Life." It refers to the idea of using technology to create a surveillance network that is controlled and monitored by the people themselves, rather than some overseeing institution. The expression has been used to refer to the ubiquity of social media, and the trend of individual users to record each other's bad behaviour (or even just perceived bad behaviour) in order to expose the person involved to the scrutiny and judgment of the masses via social media, while incurring positive social media attention, likes and 'clout' for themselves in the process. It is a certainty that any bad public behaviour you indulge in these days, particularly in the confined and intimate space of a plane cabin, will be recorded and broadcast by somebody in some way. A mistake that could be so easy to make- drinking on an empty stomach, having a few too many while waiting for a delayed flight at an airport bar, taking a pill to calm your nerves and thinking it'll be okay if you have just one glass of wine- could live on in internet infamy for the rest of your life.

In just one of many such instances, a British woman named Catherine Bush was filmed screaming in the face of a flight attendant and was later escorted off the plane to the cheers of other passengers. After she received a .£5,000 bill from the airline and the video went viral, Catherine stated, "I am so ashamed of myself. There will never be an excuse to justify what happened and I take full responsibility for my actions. I took alcohol on board the aircraft when I knew I shouldn't have. I became so intoxicated I couldn't control myself." She also admitted that she had been drinking at the airport before the flight to calm her nerves.[75]

Without condoning Catherine's behaviour towards the employees, anyone who has been intoxicated to the point of irrationality and uncontrolled emotion can probably picture themselves in a comparable situation. All the more reason to stay away from booze entirely.

81. ALCOHOL MAKES YOU WASTE YOUR EDUCATIONAL OPPORTUNITIES

I went to university in Australia. As with most things back then, I did not appreciate how little I had to pay upfront to attend my program. Which was lucky, because I had zero financial support from my family, and although I worked part-time in retail, what was left over after paying my share of the rent in the house I shared with four classmates was often just enough to buy bread or the grossest bottle of $4 plonk the Bottle-O had to offer. Since I could usually rely on housemates cooking up some extra pasta or having a spare packet of Mi-Goreng (if you know, you know) to keep me (barely) nourished, buying the wine was usually a priority.

And granted, there wasn't a lot of 'studying' required for my course. Under extreme duress, I read the plays assigned for us to analyse and the scripts we were required to perform (but often barely). It wasn't a heavily academic program by any means. Still, I look back and think, for fucks sake. If I had grown up with a broke single mother almost *anywhere* except Australia, I probably wouldn't have been able to afford to go near an institution of higher education. And I decided to use that opportunity to play Goon of Fortune and get a jump on destroying my pristine liver?

82. YOUR CAREER WILL ACCELERATE IN SOBRIETY

It's astonishing to see how quickly you can progress in your career when you untether yourself from alcohol. Considering the example of the office Christmas party, staying sober and in control in social situations involving colleagues is the only way to ensure you maintain professionalism. Let someone else photocopy their ass. Being around alcohol and not partaking shows dignity, restraint, and good judgment. Regarding your career, you want your work to be what people talk about, not your shenanigans.

Sobriety brings what feels like an endless reserve of energy. You'll wonder where it all came from. As your ability to focus improves, you'll see the encouraging effects on your work. Just as your employers and colleagues noticed your half-arsery, they'll observe the change in you. It will enable you to cultivate stronger professional relationships. You may even find you like your job, or that at least find certain aspects of it enjoyable, when you're not focused on just making it through the day without chundering into the garbage can next to your desk.

Achieving sobriety allowed me to come to the realization that I was fighting against my true calling- a successful career as an actress was not what my soul was meant for. Going through the process of healing and staying sober helped me understand that my insecurities from childhood drove my desire to become a famous actress. Once I eliminated alcohol from my life, I had the time, energy, and resources to explore other opportunities. It took me two decades of working to finally discover the career that gives me purpose and wakes me up with enthusiasm each day. I doubt I would have ever found it if I hadn't quit drinking.

So if you're feeling stuck in your current career, sobriety may be just what you need to bring about a significant change.

83. BEING SOBER WILL HELP YOU UNDERSTAND THE MEANING OF LIFE (I'M KIDDING. BUT IT MAY BRING YOU CLOSER)

Even if we've buried it under layers of mimetic desire and superficial goals, I believe that there is a yearning for a life beyond just 'going through the motions' in every person alive. An urge to understand why we're here and what the ultimate purpose of our existence is. Many people search for meaning and fulfilment in religion and philosophy, or seek it in higher education, or find it in charity work and acts of service to others. Many more of us, however, hide from the bigger questions by filling our days with temporary, feel-good, short-lived distractions. Junk food, social media and trash TV binges, pointless celebrity gossip and what I call the 'bullshit of the day', and of course, big nights out and the subsequent chaos they can wreak on a life.

84. SOBRIETY IS THE SUREST PATH TO SELF-KNOWLEDGE

I remind myself daily that internally chastising myself over how many hours I've wasted is futile. The best I can do is the best any of us can do; indeed, the only thing we *can* do is move forward. If you're reading this, you're still alive. There's still time to be enjoyed with a sense of presence. There's still time to meditate, practice sitting quietly with yourself, and connect to the feeling of contentment that lies behind the bullshit of the mind.

There is a still, quiet space within you that is okay with everything. This part of you is capable of experiencing something resembling peace because it knows it is a small manifestation of something much larger than your addictions, appetites, petty grievances, and ego.

This part of you acknowledges and understands how truly and wonderfully weird it is to have been born a human. It marvels at it. It thinks the whole thing is fascinating.

There is still time to contact the part of you that resides underneath your bullshit. There is always time.

85. ALCOHOL TURNED ME INTO A MEGA BITCH

I'm not ashamed to admit it, as it's an essential part of the healing process - I could be a right bitch when I was drunk. Alcohol brought out my own insecurities and turned them against others to try and protect my own drunken ego/false sense of self. It wasn't fair, it wasn't right, and I would probably fall into the bad cunt category by the end of the night (along with Karen).

Acting like a bad cunt comes with a level of anxiety, fear, angst and learning to shut off emotionally to protect your own ego. Those feelings are ten times worse when you can't remember what you did and said the night before and your stomach is in knots waiting for that message to say "You ok hun? You were completely maggot last night". It was almost a weekly (and even bi-weekly) event by the end of my drinking days.

The peace and serenity that going to bed sober does for your mind, body, and soul is revolutionary. Yes, I can still act like a bitch from time to time, but a big part of that inner healing was forgiving myself, learning to say sorry when I have done wrong and living life with a level of maturity that puts me in the driving seat. Sobriety allowed me to drop that toxic bitch that would usually surface when I started on the tequila shots (like, every time).

And you figure out something monumental in sobriety - you say "sorry" a LOT LESS than when you were drinking!

The other part of sobriety is that I don't waste my energy trying to belittle or bitch about other people. A big part of the 12-step program, was taking ownership of my own happiness. Moaning and belittling are side effects of drinking culture, primarily fuelled by a group of people, all drinking to forget about the week they just had. With that comes a room full of resentments, and it's a toxic environment to be around. You only need to have drunk with work colleagues on a Thursday night to see that in action.

When you shift your focus onto your own healing and away from bitching about other people to cover up your own insecurities and unhappiness - good shit happens fast!

One question I ask myself each time I start seeing myself moan or belittle someone (I'm not perfect) - what am I lacking that I need to moan or belittle that person? You soon head down a rabbit hole and come back out a more humble and grateful human because of it.

86. TRUST ME, YOU'LL FEEL SO MUCH BETTER BEING IN CONTROL

I used to think I loved getting 'loose' and hammered, but years into sobriety, the idea of not being in complete control of my actions horrifies me.

Taking back control has enabled me to get closer to being the person I want to be. Suppose I feel awkward or uncomfortable in a social situation. Rather than just throwing back drinks until I feel 'good', I'm now equipped to look at the situation critically and ask myself what may need to change. Am I spending time with the right people? Do I have unchecked issues with my self-worth and self-esteem that I may want to talk to my therapist about? Why do I not feel okay just being myself? This self-knowledge will ultimately make you the best version of yourself, as tedious as it can be in the moment.

And it is tedious. Oh god, there's pretty much nothing worse than being forced to feel your feelings of awkwardness, insecurity and anxiety after years of suppressing them. At first, it may feel almost unbearable to sit with your sober self in a social situation, naked (hopefully only metaphorically) and afraid. But it gets easier.

With practice, you will grow to feel comfortable participating in conversations and meeting new people without the artificial leg-up that alcohol gives you. This will increase your confidence and help you discover you never needed that dose of liquid courage. You'll grow in confidence and esteem in your mind, making you more appealing to others. It's so worth the temporary discomfort. I can tell you that with absolute conviction.

87. SOBRIETY ENABLES YOU TO FORM NEW AND HEALTHY HABITS

It takes just 90 days to form a new habit. This may seem daunting, but in the scheme of life, think about how fast

90 days go. In AA, newcomers are advised to attend 90 meetings in the first 90 days to cement this habit. This is more doable than ever, given the previously discussed ubiquity of online sessions.

Plus, you can use the 90-day term to implement healthy habits in place of drinking. This could be taking a half-hour walk every day for 90 days. Or journaling a couple of pages every day for 90 days. Or meditating for five minutes, every day for 90 days. Or taking a break from online shopping for 90 days. One healthy habit begets another. As time passes, and you find it's easier to do these things, your motivation will increase and you'll want to make more positive changes in your life.

Unfortunately, and you'll fucking hate me for saying this, meditation works really well as a healthy sober activity. If you're one of those people who pictures meditation as something you need a $5000 rose quartz crystal throne from that new age hippy shop in order to do, please be assured that you don't need any of that shite. Meditation is *just breathing*. You don't have to spend a cent to do it. Honestly, you don't even need a quiet place. You can meditate anywhere.

For instance, I live in a very old and noisy apartment building. My upstairs neighbours are forever engaged in some combination of sprinting laps, hammering things into the floor, and practising that wrestling move where someone leaps from the very top of the ropes and the full force of their entire body weight lands with a thud that seems to shake the continent. My downstairs neighbour is an aspiring music producer, so enough said. The building is by a busy main road, and the sound of traffic is a constant racket of screeching near-misses and car horns. But since all you have to do in order to meditate is close your eyes and breathe, it doesn't matter. Practicing finding stillness and mental quiet amid all the noise of life will make you even better at it, even more chill. There are a few ways to get started on doing this. The most important thing is to focus entirely on the breath. Just the action of the breath. If your mind starts to wander, and of course it will, don't beat yourself up. Just bring it back to focusing on the breath, as quickly but as gently as you can. Go easy on yourself. You can begin by:

- Counting breaths: Sit or lie down in a comfortable position and close your eyes. Inhale through your nose for a count of four, hold your breath for a count of four, and then exhale through your nose for a count of four. Repeat this process, making sure to focus on the counting and the sensation of the breath moving in and out of your body. This is the most straightforward mindful breathing exercise I have found, and you can do it anywhere without drawing any attention to yourself (for instance, when you're at a party and yet another person offers to grab you a drink!)

- Belly breathing: Sit with one hand on your chest and the other on your belly. Take a deep breath in through your nose, letting your belly fill with air and pushing your hand on your belly out. Hold your breath for a few seconds, then slowly exhale through your mouth, letting your belly deflate. Repeat for several minutes, focusing only on the sensation of the breath moving in and out of your body.

You'd be amazed how often you hold your breath in life, or at least fail to breathe deeply. Nothing is as calming and centring as a full and conscious breath.

88. SOBRIETY ENABLES YOU TO CULTIVATE MINDFULNESS

There are many other ways to incorporate the practice of mindfulness into your life. One of my favorites is to take a phone-free walk. For me, this means that while I still have my phone with me physically in case of emergencies, I don't look at or engage with it unless absolutely necessary.

Initially, I found this incredibly challenging. My walks used to represent yet another way to distract myself. I'd crank up the music or a podcast into my headphones and charge along, far more involved in the thing I was projecting into my mind than in the world around me. I realized that, all day long, I was just pumping my mind full of noise. I decided to see what would happen if I treated my daily walks as not another thing to get done as quickly as possible and while incurring the maximum amount of distraction, but rather as something to savour, as an end in themselves.

And at first, walking around my neighbourhood and the nearby park without piping entertainment directly into my skull was interminably dull. I was still charging through, walking as quickly as usual, just trying to get it over with. But I soon realized the key to what I was looking for was in slowing down. I lessened my pace, took deep breaths, and tried to actually become present. To feel the air on my arms and legs, to notice the various scents wafting through the air, to listen to each seperate bird-song. After so much of my life spent feeling like my mind and body were separate entities, to experience them together was a revelation. This is all mindfulness is. Feeling all of yourself, right there, in the space you are in.

And becoming mindless through excessive alcohol use, as was the case every weekend in my drinking days, is the polar opposite of mindfulness.

So do you want to be mindful or mindless? The choice is yours.

89. SOBER APPS HAVE NEVER BEEN MORE CONVENIENT

I'm a personal user of the NOMO App. NOMO allows you to create your sobriety clock for whatever you may be dealing with. My first clock was for alcohol, naturally, but I've since created clocks to help track my progress with cutting down on social media usage, and for eliminating my time-sucking propensity for watching idiotic videos on Youtube. I don't know if you've noticed, but us addictive personality types tend to replace one 'drug' with another. We quit drinking, and start heading for the fridge when we have an uncomfortable feeling instead. We erase our social media accounts, only to wind up spending every moment of the day scrolling obscure Reddit forums instead. NOMO helps me keep track of the number of days it's been since I've indulged any or all of my vices. I'm proud to say I've never had to hit reset on the Alcohol clock. The 'not fucking around on the internet' clock gets reset daily. Look, I'm trying my best.

90. SOBER DATING HAS NEVER BEEN MORE CONVENIENT

If you'd asked me what my idea of 'dating' was in my twenties, I would have said, "Getting drunk early, rolling home with a guy and hoping he texts me after." As I've said, there's NOTHING wrong with rolling home with a person right away, but it was seldom what I would have chosen to do had I been sober. I wanted to make a genuine connection. Alcohol robbed me of my agency, and I didn't think I had a choice. The idea of going on a date sober was nightmarish, out of the question entirely.

Another vital life lesson that sobriety showed me - happiness is an inside job and jumping from relationship to relationship is just another addiction - codependency.

Until I got sober, I went from relationship to relationship that all centered around alcohol. You will never meet your true self or your partner's true self if you are drunk while enjoying your downtime together. Alcohol changes people - and in my experience, it has never improved a single relationship.

If you are nervous about sober dating - wait until you are happy within yourself - you won't find what you are looking for in another relationship. To prove it, I have the 'multiple failed relationships fuelled by co-dependency and a lack of self-worth t-shirt'.

That happiness will then filter into the world and the people around you, and you WILL find the right person for you.

Side note: It's still a numbers game, so be prepared to go full pelt into dating, then go through a phase where you delete all the apps, do loads of dates again, delete the apps, become a nun, reinstall all the apps and then finally find someone or finally buy those kittens you've been eyeing up that whole time. Most importantly, have fun flaunting that new sober self with pride, confidence and sex appeal that you never had after five Espresso Martinis, ripped tights and the coordination of a one-legged horse.

Connecting via a sober app is one way to ensure the person you're on a date with feels just as raw as you. I haven't personally used any of these but the ladies in my AA meeting recommend them (over and above the 13 steppers that plague some meetings - another google opportunity).

Some sober dating apps include:

- Loosid

- Clean and Sober Love

- Sober Singles Date

- I Am Sober

- Meet Mindful

Or just use "normal" dating apps and be clear about what you want from your profile e.g. I am looking for a non-drinker, 6ft plus (sorry small guys), no children, has their own house, enjoys reading self-help and fiction books, into playing sports and so on. Equally, if you don't know what you want yet, go on dates and find out from all the car crash ones you will attend what it is you don't want (which will lead you to what you do want!). I am a big believer in manifestation, and you will receive what you put out to the world (eventually!).

Good luck.

91. NON-ALCOHOLIC OPTIONS HAVE NEVER BEEN MORE VARIED AND DELICIOUS

I'm at the stage of sobriety where I feel entirely comfortable nursing a soda or water. Still, it's understandable that you may wish to have a drink that more closely resembles what the people around you are imbibing, particularly if you're new to sobriety. Depending on the people you're around, it can also help you avoid questions you may not like answering about why you're not drinking (for help with that, might I refer you to my other book - 101 Ways To Say I Quit Drinking Alcohol Without It Being Awkward (Sort Of).

There are, of course, mocktails, popular ones being the Shirley Temple, the Virgin Mary, and the Virgin Mojito. With a virgin version of your favorite drink, you can enjoy whatever tactile pleasure you derived from holding that particular glass and tasting those distinct flavours while keeping your pants on.

And let's not discount the placebo effect; strangely enough, a virgin cocktail now puts me in the same cheerful, relaxed mood as my first cocktail of the night used to. And I've never blown up my entire life because I accidentally had too much sugar (but the night is young!)

92. MORE AND MORE PEOPLE ARE JOINING YOU IN THE JOY OF SOBRIETY

People are increasingly waking up to the lies we've been fed as a society. Young people are incensed about the mishandling of the climate crisis at the hands of governments worldwide. They are starting to understand how social media has damaged their mental health. And they are realising that they don't need alcohol to enjoy themselves and to be 'grown up'.

Generation Z, also known as 'Zoomers' or 'Gen Z', generally have a more cautious approach to alcohol consumption than previous generations. According to various studies, members of Gen Z drink less frequently and in smaller quantities than earlier generations, like millennials. According to the UK's largest recent study of drinking behaviours, 16-to-25-

year-olds were the most likely to be sober or 'sober curious', with 26% not drinking, compared to 55-to-74-year-olds, only 15% of whom didn't drink. In the United States, a study found that the percentage of college-age Americans who are teetotal has risen from 20% to 28% in a decade.[76]

In general, Gen-Z are more risk-averse than previous generations. This may be attributable, in some degree, to the fact that they grew up with the world's information at their fingertips. They have a fluency in the online world that enables them to find and connect with any community that interests them, including the sober community. Conversely, they may also have seen peers, and friends have to face disciplinary action in school and at their jobs due to their drunken antics ending up online, which has made them more cautious about partaking.

Imagine how soul-destroying it would be if THAT video went viral and you were the forever drunken meme. Don't be THAT meme.

93. IT'S EASIER THAN EVER BEFORE TO CHECK OUT A MEETING (AA OR OTHERWISE)

As much as in-person connection should be valued and cherished, attending your first meeting in the flesh can be a very intimidating experience. When I attended my first meeting, it felt like everybody knew each other, and I was quite intimidated. It took me some time to overcome my social anxiety, and to come back, and to try a variety of different meetings in different locations. What I learned is that every group is completely different. Some will have their cliques and their hierarchies. This is what happens naturally when people gather, especially over extended periods of time. The wonderful thing is there are so many meetings. They're an ever-changing, evolving entity. If one doesn't feel like your scene, try out another. One option now that was not common when I first got sober was the opportunity to attend a virtual meeting.

Although you can still feel social anxiety on Zoom, there is something decidedly less intimidating about trying out a new meeting when you can do it from the comfort of your home. You can hit up virtual meetings all day until you find one you like. No petrol money or train fare required! Besides, we all know that interacting on Zoom is inherently awkward (that lag!), so your particular awkwardness will probably go unnoticed.

My path led me into the rooms of AA, but you don't have to follow my path. There are plenty of alternatives to AA that are just as successful, SMART Recovery being an alternative, but with so many new sober communities - you are likely to find your own tribe. Just make sure that you start going to something, somewhere, with some people who have been through what you are going through - positive changes happen fast when you are in a supportive group who have walked the path you are about to embark on.

If you are looking for a great place to start, you can join the supportive Sober On A Drunk Planet Community (www.soberonadrunkplanet.com/community).

94. YOU ARE FAR FROM ALONE.

One question that often comes up for the newly sober or sober curious is, what will my social life actually look like without booze?

Suppose you're among the many people who live for your after-work drink, boozy Friday and Saturday nights, and Sunday mimosas or a Sunday Sesh at the pub. In that case, you may wonder if you will even *have* a social life. A meeting/community is a great place to begin finding sober people to connect with. Alternatively, you can take the plunge and invite someone you'd typically drink with for a coffee, a hike, or a movie. It may surprise you how cool they are with doing something besides getting pissed.

If you don't feel the connection is there without booze, you have the time and mental space to invest in friendships with the people you don't need to drink to be around. My social circle shrunk significantly when I quit drinking, but the friendships I have and maintain today are so much more fulfilling than the connections I used to make.

95. YOU CAN USE YOUR EXPERIENCES FOR GOOD

When you discover the joy of sobriety, one of the things that may develop from your newfound sense of purpose, and all the free time you suddenly have, is a desire to help others and impart some of the wisdom and experience you've gained. Many sober people become accredited drug and alcohol abuse counsellors through one of the many certificate programs available worldwide. Many of these courses do not require a college or university education, and they offer a practical component that enables you to gain hands-on experience in counselling as part of your training.

There is also writing, of course. Unlike taking a class, writing is free. It enables you to make sense and meaning out of your own experience, and ultimately to connect with others. Yes, many people are already writing about alcohol abuse and their experiences with sobriety, but so what? There is a hell of a lot of us who've struggled with this and who continue to struggle with it, more than you can possibly imagine. Your work might reach somebody at the precise moment that they need to read it. You could be the final push somebody needs to quit drinking. What you write may be the thing that encourages somebody else to stay the course of sobriety and not give up.

I will read the stories of people who've struggled with alcoholism all day. It reminds me that we are all connected, and that humans are fundamentally more alike than we are different. It is an isolating experience to feel like you're the only person among your friends who can't just have a casual drink. There is a lot of shame associated with binge drinking and alcohol abuse, and the stories of others always remind me that I'm not alone.

There are so many options. You can publish on Medium, start your own Substack newsletter, or pen a WordPress blog. Create your own book series on Amazon! Even if no one reads it (and somebody will, because so many people are going through the same thing you are), it's a cathartic experience. And by the time you finish writing it, you'll be so bored of yourself and your story that you'll be well and truly ready to move on to the next stage of your life, fortified in your sobriety. You never know what it is about your personal experience that may be the thing somebody else needs to hear.

96. BECOMING SOBER ALLOWS YOU TO EMBRACE 'JOMO'

Reframe, reframe, reframe. It's all about your mental concepts. You don't need to have FOMO. You know exactly what you're missing out on. Potentially catastrophic, life-altering health effects. Increased risk of harm to others and self. Antisocial behaviour. All of the above considered, are you really missing those nights out because of the few times that something fun happened? I promise you can still have fun sober; I've done it plenty of times. If you find yourself in your newfound sobriety experiencing FOMO, here are a few strategies:

- Mute the Insta/Snapchat/Tiktok whatever stories of your party-hard friends. You don't need to see the highlight reel of their night out right now. You know it's bullshit and they spent half the night crying in the bathroom anyway.

- Retrain your brain. Whenever you think how much 'fun' it would be to be at the bar, think of your most abjectly humiliating drunken experience. Think of it every time you feel that twinge of FOMO. Drown your thoughts in reminiscing about your own indignity.

• Fill the time with an activity you've always wanted to try. If you've thought of yourself as something of a writer, start writing. Try free-writing. It's unbelievable just how many creative people swear by the practice of waking up and writing three pages of whatever comes into their minds, every single day. Julia Cameron popularised this exercise in her seminal book 'The Artists Way'. Write anything that pops into your head, no matter how banal, inconsequential, or petty. Write about how much you hate the exercise, need to poop, and how annoying it is when your upstairs neighbour does whatever the fuck they're constantly doing up there. It doesn't matter. Do this every day for a month. I promise you, it will change something within you. You will gain clarity. If nothing else, you can read your work later and laugh at all the ridiculous things that cross your mind at any given moment.

Sobriety allows you to embrace the 'Joy of Missing Out' (JOMO) and see every area of your life improve as a result. You might get itchy feet on a Thursday night thinking "I wonder how much fun all my work colleagues are having without me" - the truth is, nobody cares. They are doing all the things you want to avoid, and seeing them all the following day, hungover and weary-eyed, confirms that you made the right choice. In time, you will see a clear pattern emerge - you really aren't missing out on anything.

Saying NO can be your best tool for rocket launching your own self-growth and happiness - so use it.

97. RECOVERY ENABLES YOU TO RECOGNISE CODEPENDENT RELATIONSHIPS AND MAKE HEALTHIER CHOICES

When you begin navigating friendships and relationships as a sober person, you do so with a vastly increased sense of self-awareness. The 'soul-searching' you do in the beginning stages of sobriety will enable you to recognise destructive mental patterns within yourself and patterns in your relationships. You may realize that a friendship or relationship has a codependent aspect and decide to make a change.

Sobriety enables you to set healthier boundaries. Rather than reeling from one chaotic relationship to another, you will have the lucidity and perspective to consider what it is you really want. As I said earlier, I often found myself having drunken one-night stands when what I was really seeking was a relationship or connection with a particular person. One evening of feeling sexually desired felt like 'enough', even though it was a poor substitute for what I wanted. I settled for such superficial connections over and over because I didn't have the self-worth to believe that anyone would be interested in me when I was sober and not offering myself to them immediately. Again, there's nothing wrong with casual sex and one-night stands, as long as it's you in the driver's seat deciding to partake and not the influence of alcohol.

98. SOBRIETY ENABLES YOU TO REBUILD YOUR RELATIONSHIPS

As discussed earlier, sobriety tends to weed out certain relationships and friendships. Some of the connections you have may fail to survive. Some may evolve. Those that remain will be enhanced exponentially. They will benefit from the following:

- Improved communication. No more bottling shit up and letting rip as soon as you're a few drinks in. No more hashing out the petty issues of your relationship in front of your uncomfortable friends over drinks. I can almost guarantee fewer arguments once you get sober.

- Increased trust. It's a lot easier to have confidence in a relationship with someone who isn't continually losing their phone and confused about how they managed to get home. Can you trust your partner when they go out drinking a psychoactive drug (alcohol) that also lowers their inhibitions? I might have trust issues, but seeing plenty of marriages and relationships fail because of a drunken mistake makes you sceptical.

- Greater emotional intimacy. More time spent with your partner or friends while sober enables you to get to know them, as does bonding over activities that aren't drinking at the pub.

99. SOBRIETY IS BETTER THAN ANY JUICE CLEANSE OR DIET

What happens to your body when you stop drinking alcohol? As we've discussed, detoxification can be physically gruelling and even dangerous. Again, we must reiterate that if you have reason to believe you have a severe physical dependence on alcohol, you must consult a medical professional before stopping.

If you don't think you have a severe dependence, but you find yourself experiencing hallucinations, delirium tremens (DTs), seizures or other concerning symptoms in the first few days drink-free, consult a medical professional immediately.

After one week without alcohol, your risk of seizures decreases, and your risk of cardiovascular issues declines. Your liver also starts to repair itself. Phew!

After six weeks of abstinence from alcohol, your brain mass will increase by an average of 2%. You will likely feel more positive overall.[77] You may notice increased energy and stamina, that your skin and eyes start clear up, and that you've dropped a few pounds. Keep it up! It only gets better. No starving yourself and drinking weird juice that makes you sit on the loo all day required.

100. QUITTING ALCOHOL ENABLES YOU TO BEGIN THE VIRTUOUS CYCLE

Good habits beget other good habits. We know the vicious cycles of alcohol abuse: working jobs we despise, blowing the entirety of our paycheques on partying because we feel like we've earned it through our misery and deserve it. Spending a couple of days hungover or coming down, never able to progress because our performance at work doesn't rise above mediocrity, and why would we care anyway, since we hate this job? Bundling up our true passions, our actual dreams, whether that be for starting our own business or just taking some classes, shoving those dreams into some dark corner of our mind where we can ignore them because we 'don't have time' or 'it's all too hard.' Or convincing ourselves that we'll get to them eventually; meanwhile the years seem to pass by faster and faster.

Then there's the virtuous cycle you'll find yourself in sobriety. Waking up clear-headed on a Saturday or Sunday morning and realising you have the entire day before you. Making it out the door for one of those morning walks your fit friend constantly nags you to go on. Having the motivation to clean your apartment or crack open that book that's been gathering dust on your nightstand for a year instead of scrolling your phone in front of Love Island all day, dreading Monday morning already. Your time is yours again. You may wonder what the hell you're even going to do with it. Embrace boredom. Embrace the day unfolding before you. Soon, you'll have so many things you want to do that you won't know where to begin.

101. ONE DAY IT WILL BE SO EASY

I don't even think about drinking anymore. I mean, I thought about it a lot while working on this book. But before that, almost never. It's just no longer part of my life. I don't crave it. I don't miss it. I don't have to read and re-read the above reasons to remind myself of the Joy of Missing Out. I've been living it, and eventually, you will too. I've reached a place of complete and total comfort with carrying around a bottle of water or a soft drink at a party. No one really bothers to ask, but I'm at the stage of 'fuck it' self-assurance where if anybody does, I just tell them I'm an alcoholic. Sometimes, disarming honesty is the best course of action. Nobody argues with that. I did write a book of 101 Ways to Say 'I Don't Drink Alcohol', which is available for you to refer to if you're feeling like a sillier or more flirtatious response. You may get to the point where you don't feel you need to explain yourself at all, and you can smile and say "No thanks", and walk away if the person trying to get you a drink presses the issue. There's nothing wrong with a mysterious shrug or a wink as you say "Nah, I'm good." It's your life and your body now!

And as your body and mind adjust and any withdrawal symptoms start to diminish, the urge to imbibe will grow dimmer and dimmer as every area of your life goes from strength to strength. That's when you realize, like everyone in sobriety, that you wished you had found it sooner.

CONCLUSION

Congratulations on making it through to the end of these 101 harrowing reasons why you should give up alcohol! I brought this book to you with the best of intentions, and through researching and writing it, I learned so much I didn't know about alcohol and its destructive effects. I really hope you've learned something too! Again, I'm no expert in anything, but my aim in collating and presenting all the terrors of drinking in this way was mainly to encourage you to start or stay on the path. Whether you're sober-curious or further along the road, motivation is always necessary.

My intention is not to pass judgment on those who choose to imbibe. Do I think my friends, family and husband would all be happier and healthier if they were sober? Of course. Do I want them to live as long as possible? Absolutely. But I choose to live and let live when it comes to my real life. You, on the other hand, I'm allowed to lecture. You bought this book, or somehow procured it, and you read it this far. Thank you, by the way. I know there are a lot of texts on sobriety out there (including, perhaps, the one you're going to write yourself!) Throughout the course of writing this, I experienced a lot of self-doubt and the persistent question of "why does anyone need my take on this?" And the answer is that they don't, but I pissed away my potential and prospects in my younger years and rambling about my trauma is all I've got to make myself significant in the world. Just kidding, I want to help people and sobriety allowed me to re-connect with my childhood passion for writing. And here we are!

Two powerful re-caps that bring all the 101 reasons of why you need to quit drinking full circle:

1) Alcohol is like negative equity - all the hard work and money you pump into alcohol, it ends up taking all your initial investment of time, energy, money, relationships and more! Sobriety allows you to gain all that back and more - in new and exciting ways.

2) Don't be a Karen.

There is so much positive change to be had when you become sober. If you're somehow still not convinced (come on, man), indulge me in the briefest of recaps:

- Your liver, heart, and brain, the miraculous organs that each have their role in keeping you alive and well, are so heavily taxed by your alcohol consumption. They are essential; booze is not. The long-term health ramifications are potentially so devastating, so numerous, that it would seem utterly bonkers to someone who'd grown up in a world without alcohol that we would do this to ourselves!

- By quitting drinking as early as possible, you can significantly reduce your risk of developing a wide range of health problems, such as liver disease, heart disease, and cancer. You will also have more energy, and feel better overall. Things you perhaps didn't even conceive of as related to your alcohol consumption may improve, such as your skin, and your irritable bowels!

- Your mental health will improve. You will no longer spend days of your life in the throes of 'Hangxiety', spiralling over what you said or did the night before, whether you're going to lose your job because you fucked off work yet again, and the fact that you spent your rent money on bottle service. By removing the fog and influence of alcohol, you will gain a clarity and presence of mind that enables you to deal with what you may have been trying to drown out with excessive drinking. You'll have to face up to some shit, a process that, while painful, will ultimately lead you to your best chance of contentment and true happiness.

- Your relationships will get better. No more starting inane, drunken fights with your partner over the most minor infractions or perceived slights. No more unsatisfying, perhaps even hazardous sexual encounters with people you wouldn't even consider in the cold light of day. No more rambling 'deep and meaningfuls' with bar rando's you won't remember or recognise the next time you see them. Sobriety will make you more present in conversation and lead you to develop more profound and lasting connections with the people around you.

- Sobriety will lead you to greater effectiveness in your work. If you're eager to progress in the job you're currently in, it will be much easier to do so when you aren't nursing hangovers at your desk. Your colleagues and bosses will notice the uptick in your enthusiasm and focus, and you may find your prospects and opportunities growing beyond what you envisaged!

- You'll reap the financial benefits. Big nights out are insanely expensive. When you get sober from alcohol, you break the cycle you may have fallen into of working for the weekend, and then blowing your paycheque on an essentially empty 'good time'. This is the cycle that has imprisoned so many in jobs they are deeply unsatisfied with. By cutting out the nights out, you give yourself the time, energy, mental space and financial bandwidth to pursue a different path, or a course of study that enables you to find a more fulfilling position.

- You'll find yourself becoming more present, mindful and even spiritual (if you're into that sort of thing). No matter how you conceive of a 'higher power', whether you believe in the existence of a God or an all-encompassing Universe, sobriety enables you to connect to this in a greater way.

- Being sober enables you to achieve greater emotional stability. The de-inhibiting and de-regulating effects of alcohol on your moods can lead to problems in your personal and professional life. When you cut it out, you take back control and give yourself the gift of enhanced emotional maturity and resilience.

- Your sleep will improve, as the effects of drinking on your REM sleep will disappear. You'll have more energy and a vastly improved mood throughout the day.

- You'll regain control of your life. Frequent heavy drinking leads to the sensation of your life not being your own and the feeling that you're just careening from one chaotic episode to another. In sobriety, it is all up to you, and you can shape the rest of your life in whichever way you choose.

- In sobriety, you will remove, or at least significantly decrease, the possibility of doing something that could hurt or even kill another person. No more of your addled brain attempting to convince you that you "drive better when you've had a few." No more drunken rage, no chance that you'll be involved in a brawl or make a split-second decision that irrevocably changes the course of your life or somebody else's life. You're in the driver's seat (sober).

At first, it may seem as though the whole world is chugging beers and popping champagne (or doing that weird knife thing to open the bottle) while you're practising saying no, but be assured, even people in the hedonistic world of show business are consciously resisting the lure of alcohol. So if you are still not convinced (I have tried my best to this point) the wisdom of these sober celebrities may be what you need to hear:

"Being in recovery has given me everything of value that I have in my life. Integrity, honesty, fearlessness, faith, a relationship with God, and most of all, gratitude. It's given me a beautiful family and an amazing career. I'm under no illusions where I would be without the gift of alcoholism and the chance to recover from it." - *Rob Lowe, an actor with more than 25 years of sobriety under his belt.*

"All I knew is if I was continuing to go down the road I was, I would either end up dead or, like, doing something really, really stupid. It was always something I was very scared of, but I think I needed that community."- *Actress and model Cara Delevigne talking about her involvement in the 12-step program.*

"The drinking thing for me was a constant, like, 'You cannot change. You are weak and incapable of doing what's best for you. You keep thinking you will master this thing, and it's getting the better of you. " - *Drew Barrymore, actress, producer and TV host.*

"Now I don't drink, and this is why: I was belligerent and said a bunch of s–t I shouldn't have said on the red carpet after that. I'm sure I got in a lot of trouble for what I said ... I don't remember why but I know that I did." - *Megan Fox, actress.*

"It's really hard (being sober) because especially being young, there's that stigma of 'you're no fun. It's like, 'Honey, you can call me a lot of things, but I know that I'm fun."- *Miley Cyrus, singer and actress.*

"I wanted to understand myself because I didn't even realize how much I was drinking and how much I was suppressing. I thought it was making me brave, I thought it was making me confident, and it was actually the complete opposite, it was silencing me." - *Jessica Simpson, former singer and actress.*

"I have completed treatment for alcohol addiction; something I've dealt with in the past and will continue to confront. I want to live life to the fullest and be the best father I can be."- *Ben Affleck, Oscar-winning director and actor.*

"During that time I avoided looking in the mirror, because I didn't like the person who was looking back at me. To be honest, there were times I thought I wouldn't survive. I used to have a lot of problems. Amongst others I drank too much, so I joined Alcoholics Anonymous to get and stay sober."- *Supermodel Naomi Campbell.*

"It took me a long time, a long time disappointing everyone who cared about me, culminating in a terrible DUI where I could have killed somebody. I hit rock bottom." - *John Stamos, actor.*[78]

"Thinking about not drinking forever was very scary, but once I did, it wasn't hard anymore because I had all of these miracles happen that let me know I was on exactly the right path." - *Lana Del Rey, singer-songwriter.*

"Getting sober was the single bravest thing I've ever done, and will ever do, in my life. Being courageous enough to acknowledge it privately with my family and friends. Working really hard at solidifying it, getting support around it, and being healthy. And then talking about it publicly. That is the single greatest accomplishment of my life." - *Jamie Lee Curtis, actress and Oscar winner.*

"Sometimes you can only find Heaven by slowly backing away from Hell." - *Carrie Fisher, actress and author of acclaimed autobiographical humor book 'Wishful Drinking'.*

"I don't drink or do drugs anymore. I realized I wasn't going to live up to my potential, and that scared the hell out of me. I thought, 'Wow, I'm actually gonna ruin my life. I'm really gonna ruin it.'" - *Bradley Cooper, actor (whose breakthrough role was, incidentally, in 'The Hangover') and director.*

"I've been the lead in movies, on television shows and nominated for Emmy. But the best thing I can say about me is that people who can't stop drinking come up to me and say, 'Can you help me?' And I can say, 'Yes.'" - *Matthew Perry, actor.*

"The problem of alcohol is, it's just too easy. It's everywhere. At least hard drugs, you have to have a dealer. All I know is, I could feel its presence in an ominous, daunting way that was preventing me from being my higher self." – *Ben Harper, singer-songwriter.*[79]

"The word 'recovery' means that we recover the person we were intended to be" - *Russell Brand, actor, comedian, podcaster, author and sober sage, with my person favorite quote on sobriety of all time.*[80]

With this in mind, who do you believe you were intended to be? You're alive (I assume) and reading this, which means there is still time. You may falter. You may slip. But this is part of the process. Starting sobriety is highly encouraged, especially if you could relate to most of this book, take it as a sign, a kick up the backside or just enough fuel to get to the gym, join that AA meeting, meet up with that sober group and stop being a slave to alcohol.

From the seven years I have been sober, I still haven't met anyone who says they regret giving up alcohol. Sobriety really does deliver everything that alcohol promises - at least give it a try (especially if you relate to most of this book!).

If you have enjoyed reading 101 Reasons, I would be grateful if you could spare 60 seconds to leave a short review on Amazon using the next page, even if it's just

196

a few sentences. It helps keep the Mulberry collection alive.

Thanks for reading.

LEAVE A REVIEW

If you have enjoyed this book, I would be extremely grateful if you could leave a review on Amazon - even if it's just a few sentences long. The review will go a long way to keeping the Mulberry collection alive - thank you.

UNITED STATES	UNITED KINGDOM
SCAN ME	SCAN ME
CANADA	REST OF WORLD
SCAN ME	SCAN ME

EXPLORE YOUR NEXT READ

WWW.SOBERONADRUNKPLANET.COM/BOOKS

A FREE GIFT FOR YOU

Just for you

SCAN ME

A FREE GIFT TO YOU

5 Sober Secrets To A Successful Sobriety
(And How To Manifest Your Dream
Handbag)

NEED SUPPORT IN YOUR JOURNEY?

WWW.SOBERONADRUNKPLANET.COM/COMMUNITY

JOIN THE EARLY REVIEW TEAM

Sign Up To Our Early Review
Team And Read Sienna's
Next Book Before Anyone
Else Does!

CITATIONS

[1] Bon Scott, Wikipedia: https://en.wikipedia.org/wiki/Bon_Scott

[2] Alcohol poisoning, Mayo Clinc: https://www.mayoclinic.org/diseases-conditions/alcohol-poisoning/symptoms-causes/syc-20354386

[3] Interrupted Memories: Alcohol-Induced Blackouts: https://www.niaaa.nih.gov/publications/brochures-and-fact-sheets/interrupted-memories-alcohol-induced-blackouts

[4] Blood Alcohol Level. Notre Dame College: https://www.notredamecollege.edu/sites/default/files/-Blood-Alcohol-Chart.pdf. Accessed 20 June 2023.

[5] NIH study finds chronic alcohol use shifts brain's control of behavior: https://www.nih.gov/news-events/news-releases/nih-study-finds-chronic-alcohol-use-shifts-brains-control-behavior

[6] Alcohol: Does it affect blood pressure? Mayo Clinic. https://www.mayoclinic.org/diseases-conditions/high-blood-pressure/expert-answers/blood-pressure/faq-20058254)

[7] High blood pressure (hypertension) - Symptoms and causes. Mayo Clinic. https://www.mayoclinic.org/diseases-conditions/high-blood-pressure/symptoms-causes/syc-20373410

[8] Alcoholic Beverage Consumption. https://ntp.niehs.nih.gov/ntp/roc/content/profiles/alcoholicbeverageconsumption.pdf

[9] Cancer Warning Labels on Alcohol Containers: A Consumer's Right to Know, a Government's Responsibility to Inform, and an Industry's Power to Thwart. https://pubmed.ncbi.nlm.nih.gov/32359059/

[10] Alcohol and Cancer | CDC. https://www.cdc.gov/cancer/alcohol/index.htm

[11] Alcohol and Cancer Risk Fact Sheet - NCI - National Cancer Institute. https://www.cancer.gov/about-cancer/causes-prevention/risk/alcohol/alcohol-fact-sheet

[12] Alcohol use: Weighing risks and benefits - Mayo Clinic. https://www.mayoclinic.org/healthy-lifestyle/nutrition-and-healthy-eating/in-depth/alcohol/art-20044551

[13] Brain Shrinkage Caused by Alcohol: Is It Reversible? https://www.verywellmind.com/cause-of-brain-shrinkage-in-alcoholics-studied-66615

[14] Alcohol's Damaging Effects On The Brain: https://pubs.niaaa.nih.gov/publications/aa63/aa63.htm

[15] Alcohol-related thiamine deficiency - Alcohol and Drug Foundation - ADF. https://adf.org.au/insights/alcohol-related-thiamine-deficiency/

[16] Thiamine deficiency, alcohol, and alcoholism. https://alcohol.addictionblog.org/thiamine-deficiency-alcohol-and-alcoholism/

[17] Wernicke-Korsakoff Syndrome | National Institute of Neurological Disorders and Stroke. https://www.ninds.nih.gov/health-information/disorders/wernicke-korsakoff-syndrome

[18] Alcoholic hepatitis - Symptoms and causes. https://www.mayoclinic.org/diseases-conditions/alcoholic-hepatitis/symptoms-causes/syc-20351388

[19] Cirrhosis - Symptoms and causes. Mayo Clinic. https://www.mayoclinic.org/diseases-conditions/cirrhosis/symptoms-causes/syc-20351487

[20] Alcohol-Related Liver Disease. Alcohol.org. https://alcohol.org/effects/alcoholic-fatty-liver-disease/

[21] Alcoholic Cardiomyopathy: Causes, Symptoms, and Diagnosis. https://www.healthline.com/health/alcoholism/cardiomyopathy

[22] Heart failure - Symptoms and causes. https://www.mayoclinic.org/diseases-conditions/heart-failure/symptoms-causes/syc-20373142

[23] Drink alcohol within the safe limits | Stroke Association. https://www.stroke.org.uk/what-is-stroke/what-can-i-do-to-reduce-my-risk/drink-less-alcohol

[24] Alcohol-Induced Pancreatitis: What is it? https://alcohol.org/comorbid/pancreatitis/

[25] Why Does Alcohol Make You Pee? https://www.healthline.com/health/why-does-alcohol-make-you-pee#effect-on-urination

[26] https://www.verywellhealth.com/how-alcohol-can-cause-bloating-4169661

[27] Dysbiosis: Test, Treatment, and More. https://www.healthline.com/health/digestive-health/dysbiosis

[28] The gut-brain connection. https://www.health.harvard.edu/diseases-and-conditions/the-gut-brain-connection

[29] Alcohol and Weight Gain Explained. https://www.health.com/weight-loss/does-alcohol-make-you-gain-weight

[30] Psoriasis and Alcohol: How Can Drinking Affect Your Symptoms? https://www.healthline.com/health/psoriasis/psoriasis-and-alcohol

[31] Does Alcohol Cause Acne? Effects of Beer, Wine, and More. https://www.healthline.com/health/beauty-skin-care/does-alcohol-cause-acne#immune-system-and-bacteria

[32] Why Alcohol Lingers On Your Breath. https://www.huffpost.com/entry/alcohol-breath_b_898103

[33] How Alcohol Affects Your Dental Health. https://www.healthline.com/health/dental-and-oral-health/what-does-alcohol-do-to-your-teeth

[34] Drinking and Your Eyes - Alcohol and Vision. https://www.verywellhealth.com/how-does-drinking-alcohol-affect-your-eyes-3421855

[35] Telogen Effluvium: Symptoms, Causes, Treatment & Regrowth.
https://my.clevelandclinic.org/health/diseases/24486-telogen-effluvium

[36] Do You Wet the Bed After a Night of Drinking?
https://health.clevelandclinic.org/adults-booze-bedwetting-heres-happens/

[37] Landon Grier: 5 Fast Facts You Need to Know.
https://heavy.com/news/landon-grier/

[38] Why Some People Get Hives From Alcohol.
https://www.soberrecovery.com/addiction/why-some-people-get-hives-from-alcohol/

[39] Peptic ulcer - Symptoms and causes.
https://www.mayoclinic.org/diseases-conditions/peptic-ulcer/symptoms-causes/syc-20354223

[40] Yeast infection (vaginal) - Symptoms and causes.
https://www.mayoclinic.org/diseases-conditions/yeast-infection/symptoms-causes/syc-20378999

[41] What Foods Can Cause a Yeast Infection?
https://www.livestrong.com/article/198027-what-foods-can-cause-a-yeast-infection/

[42] Is There a Connection Between STDs and Alcohol Use?
https://alcoholicsanonymous.com/alcohol-and-reproductive-health/stds-and-alcohol-use/

[43] Alcohol and Sleep. https://www.sleepfoundation.org/nutrition/alcohol-and-sleep

[44] Does Alcohol Kill Sperm? Learn How It Affects Sperm and Your Fertility. https://www.healthline.com/health/does-alcohol-kill-sperm-2#effect-on-male-fertility

[45] Female fertility: Why lifestyle choices count.
https://www.mayoclinic.org/healthy-lifestyle/getting-pregnant/in-depth/female-fertility/art-20045887

[46] Fetal alcohol syndrome - Symptoms and causes.
https://www.mayoclinic.org/diseases-conditions/fetal-alcohol-syndrome/symptoms-causes/syc-20352901

[47] Cognitive Impairment and Recovery.
https://pubs.niaaa.nih.gov/publications/aa53.htm

[48] Neuroplasticity.
https://www.psychologytoday.com/us/basics/neuroplasticity

[49] Recovery of neurocognitive functions following sustained abstinence after substance dependence and implications for treatment.
https://www.sciencedirect.com/science/article/abs/pii/S0272735814001196

[50] Alcohol use disorder - Symptoms and causes.
https://www.mayoclinic.org/diseases-conditions/alcohol-use-disorder/symptoms-causes/syc-20369243

[51] The Impact of Alcohol-Related Injury.
https://www.alcoholrehabguide.org/resources/medical-conditions/injury/

[52] Status Epilepticus.
https://www.hopkinsmedicine.org/health/conditions-and-diseases/status-epilepticus

[53] Alcohol Withdrawal: Symptoms, Treatment and Alcohol Detox Duration. https://www.webmd.com/mental-health/addiction/alcohol-withdrawal-symptoms-treatments

[54] Alcohol and Heart Health: Separating Fact from Fiction.
https://www.hopkinsmedicine.org/health/wellness-and-prevention/alcohol-and-heart-health-separating-fact-from-fiction

[55] Excessive Alcohol Use and Risks to Women's Health | CDC.
https://www.cdc.gov/alcohol/fact-sheets/womens-health.htm

[56] Nearly half a million more adults on antidepressants in England.
https://www.bbc.com/news/health-62094744

[57] Alcohol-Medication Interactions: Potentially Dangerous Mixes.
https://www.niaaa.nih.gov/health-professionals-communities/core-resource-on-alcohol/alcohol-medication-interactions-potentially-dangerous-mixes

[58] Diabetes and Alcohol | Effects of Alcohol on Diabetes. https://www.webmd.com/diabetes/guide/drinking-alcohol

[59] Does Alcohol Change Your Personality - How Alcohol Affects Personality. https://www.harpersbazaar.com/beauty/health/a707/does-alcohol-change-your-personality/

[60] Alcohol and Neurotransmitter Interactions. https://pubs.niaaa.nih.gov/publications/arh21-2/144.pdf

[61] List of deaths through alcohol. https://en.wikipedia.org/wiki/List_of_deaths_through_alcohol

[62] Alcohol and Neurotransmitter Interactions. https://pubs.niaaa.nih.gov/publications/arh21-2/144.pdf

[63] Dopamine: What It Is, Function & Symptoms. https://my.clevelandclinic.org/health/articles/22581-dopamine

[64] Alcohol Addiction Affects Dopamine Levels In Brain, Making It Harder To Catch A Buzz, Easier To Relapse. https://www.medicaldaily.com/alcohol-addiction-dopamine-levels-376577

[65] Is Alcohol Impacting Your Relationship? https://www.psychologytoday.com/us/blog/couples-thrive/201905/is-alcohol-impacting-your-relationship

[66] Loneliness and alcohol abuse: a review of evidences of an interpla. https://pubmed.ncbi.nlm.nih.gov/1566121/

[67] 1 in 10 People Are Fired or Disciplined After an Office Christmas Party. https://blog.jobbio.com/2018/12/10/1-in-10-people-are-fired-or-disciplined-after-an-office-christmas-party/

[68] Chasing Hope. https://dartcenter.org/content/chasing-hope?section=all

[69] Alcohol, drugs and murder: A study of convicted homicide offenders. https://www.sciencedirect.com/science/article/abs/pii/0047235290900025

[70] What Is the Connection Between Alcohol and Suicide?. https://www.verywellmind.com/alcoholics-suicide-risk-increases-with-age-63111

[71] Drug poisoning deaths in England and Wales reach record high. https://www.theguardian.com/society/2021/aug/03/drug-poisoning-deaths-in-england-and-wales-reach-record-high

[72] Australia 'one-punch' attack: First man jailed under new law. https://www.bbc.com/news/world-australia-42274932

[73] It's not just a bad hangover – this is how alcohol affects the environment. https://www.independent.co.uk/climate-change/opinion/alcohol-climate-crisis-environment-b1812946.html

[74] How Alcohol Affects Your Body Differently When You're On A Plane. https://www.huffpost.com/entry/drinking-alcohol-plane-flight-effects_l_6247588de4b0e44de9c1e9cd

[75] Woman 'sorry' after she's kicked off flight for 'trying to open plane door'. https://www.thesun.co.uk/news/18140474/woman-sorry-banned-jet2-flight/

[76] Why Gen Zers are growing up sober curious. https://www.bbc.com/worklife/article/20220920-why-gen-zers-are-growing-up-sober-curious

[77] What Happens When You Stop Drinking Alcohol? https://www.verywellmind.com/what-happens-when-you-stop-drinking-alcohol-timeline-5324861

[78] Celebrities Who Talked About Sobriety: Chrissy Teigen and More. https://www.lifeandstylemag.com/posts/celebrities-who-talked-about-sobriety-chrissy-teigen-and-more/

[79] 100 Most Inspiring Addiction Recovery Quotes. https://recovered.org/blog/100-inspiring-recovery-quotes

[80] Dua Lipa: At Your Service, Russell Brand. https://www.bbc.co.uk/programmes/p0cj45q0

Made in the USA
Monee, IL
29 August 2024

64866772R00125